KU-692-837

The Rehabilitation of People with Spinal Cord Injury

Second Edition

Shanker Nesathurai, MD, FRCP(C)
Editor

Chairman *ad interim* of Rehabilitation Medicine
Assistant Professor of Rehabilitation Medicine
Boston University School of Medicine

Chief of Rehabilitation Services
Boston Medical Center

Published 2000
ISBN # 0-632-04526-4
Library of Congress # pending publication
© 2000 Boston Medical Center
www.bumc.bu.edu / rehab

Blackwell Science, Inc.

©2000 by Boston Medical Center

Blackwell Science, Inc.

Editorial Offices:
Commerce Place, 350 Main Street, Malden, Massachusetts 02148, USA
Osney Mead, Oxford OX2 0EL, England
25 John Street, London WC1N 2BL, England
23 Ainslie Place, Edinburgh EH3 6AJ, Scotland
54 University Street, Carlton, Victoria 3053, Australia
Other Editorial Offices:
Blackwell Wissenschafts-Verlag GmbH, Kurfürstendamn 57, 10707 Berlin, Germany
Blackwell Science KK, MG Kodenmacho Building, 7-10 Kodenmacho Nihombashi,
Chuo-ku, Tokyo 104, Japan

Distributors:

USA
Blackwell Science, Inc.
Commerce Place
350 Main Street
Malden, Massachusetts 02148
(Telephone orders: 800-215-1000 or
781-388-8250; fax orders: 781-388-8270)

Australia
Blackwell Science Pty, Ltd.
54 University Street
Carlton, Victoria 3053
(Telephone orders: 03-9347-0300;
fax orders: 03-9349-3016)

Canada
Login Brothers Book Company
324 Saulteaux Crescent
Winnipeg, Manitoba, R3J 3T2
(Telephone orders: 204-837-2987)

Outside North America and Australia
Blackwell Science, Ltd.
c/o Marston Book Services, Ltd.
P.O. Box 269
Abingdon
Oxon OX14 4YN
England
(Telephone orders: 44-01235-465500;
fax orders: 44-01235-465555)

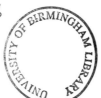

All rights reserved. No part of this book may be reproduced in any form or by any electronic or
mechanical means, including information storage and retrieval systems, without permission in
writing from the publisher, except by a reviewer who may quote brief passages in a review.
Printed in the United States of America
99 00 01 02 5 4 3 2 1

The Blackwell Science logo is a trade mark of Blackwell Science Ltd.,
registered at the United Kingdom Trade Marks Registry

Table of Contents

Notice: The indications and dosages of all drugs in this book have been recommended in the medical literature and conform to the practices of the general community. The medications described do not necessarily have specific approval by the Food and Drug Administration for use in the diseases and dosages for which they are recommended. The package insert for each drug should be consulted for use and dosage as approved by the FDA. Because standards for usage change, it is advisable to keep abreast of revised recommendations, particularly those concerning new drugs.

This book is dedicated
to my loving wife Nancy
and our precious daughter
Anne Thavam.

Introduction

A rehabilitation physician faces no greater challenge than coordinating the care of a patient with a spinal cord injury (SCI). To achieve optimal outcomes, the practitioner must understand both the biological and sociomedical issues. SCI clinicians must become adept at navigating through the arcane and complex public and private programs that may help their patients. On occasion, the programs designed to help persons with SCI have perverse incentives, which may impair social and vocational reintegration. Rehabilitation clinicians should also be cognizant of the architectural and attitudinal barriers that affect community reintegration. Spinal cord injury may not only profoundly impair the affected individual's functional independence; it also places a significant emotional and financial burden on both families and society. Despite these profound challenges, most people with SCI live satisfying and productive lives, with the support of friends and family.

For optimal outcomes, it is necessary to have a dedicated and knowledgeable team of physicians, nurses and therapists. This book is intended to provide an overview of the clinical issues for resident physicians. However, other members of the health-care team may find the monograph of interest. It provides guidelines for evaluation and management, but is by no means a comprehensive textbook. Often, the management strategies outlined reflect the practices and preferences of the contributors. As always, treatment decisions must be individualized. Many issues in SCI care have not been examined in a rigorous scientific manner. As such, the contributors hope that the readers will be inspired to organize and participate in studies that will contribute to scientific understanding.

The response to and comments about this monograph have been overwhelming. As such, this second edition contains a number of additions and revisions, including a new chapter on the pathophysiology of SCI, two new contributors, and two new illustrations.

Although care has been taken with regard to the indications, contraindications and doses of interventions, the final responsibility rests with the prescribing practitioner. The side effects of certain medications may be greater in persons with SCI. As such, the maximum recommended doses of some drugs in this monograph are lower than what is generally accepted in other populations. The readers are advised to critically review any treatment recommendations and, if necessary, refer to appropriate reference literature (e.g., Physicians' Desk Reference, American Hospital Formulary Service Drug Information Manual).

In the text, impairment of all four limbs has been categorized as *tetraplegia*, not quadriplegia. As well, skin breakdown has been labeled as *pressure ulcers* as opposed to the commonly used term decubitus ulcers. At present, tetraplegia and pressure ulcers are the preferred nomenclature.

Again, the contributors welcome the comments and criticisms of the readers. These suggestions can be incorporated into future editions.

Acknowledgments

The production and distribution of this monograph was financially supported by a National Institute on Disability and Rehabilitation Research (NIDRR) grant (H133N950014-98A) to The New England Regional Spinal Cord Injury Center (NERSCIC) at Boston Medical Center. The NERSCIC is a U.S. Department of Education-designated National Model Spinal Cord Injury System Center. The following model system's centers collaborated with the NERSCIC in the production of this monograph: University of Alabama at Birmingham, Rehabilitation Institute of Chicago, Rehabilitation Institute of Michigan, and Rancho Los Amigos Hospital. This book is being distributed gratis to junior rehabilitation medicine residents as part of NIDRR's mission of disseminating knowledge and educating health-care professionals. Additional copies are available at a nominal cost by contacting the publisher (see page 121).

This project was supported by Toby Lawrence, PT, and Joel Myklebust, PhD, project officers at NIDRR. The contributors are grateful for their guidance and assistance. In addition, the following clinicians reviewed the manuscript and provided insightful criticisms: Drs. Chunbo Cai, David Chen, Mel Glenn, Robert Krane, Radha Vijayakumar, Emilia Semenov, Karen Smith and Buck Woo and Kim Eberhart, OT. Drs. Fred Maynard and David Apple, and Ms. Leslie Hudson provided considerable telephone advice with regard to ASIA scoring. Law professor Ilene Klein kindly reviewed the section on Social Security, Medicare and Medicaid benefits. Many of their suggestions were incorporated in the final text. The authors are grateful to Scott Edwards, Patricia Regan, and Marjorie Scott for their editorial assistance. The original artwork was prepared by Edward Skawinski, Richard Francey, and Jason Laramie.

Although the contributors are gratified by the support their respective institutions have provided, the opinions and comments expressed in this monograph are those of the authors. The opinions espoused are not endorsed by any organization, agency or reviewer.

Finally, the editor would like to acknowledge the thoughtful guidance and encouragement of Dr. Allan Meyers, the research director of the NERSCIC.

Contributors

**New England Regional Spinal Cord Injury Center
at Boston Medical Center**

Dain Allred
Medical Student
Boston University School of Medicine

Amy Bjornson, MPT, ATP
Senior Physical Therapist

Susan Biener Bergman, MD
Associate Clinical Professor of Rehabilitation Medicine
Boston University School of Medicine

Stanley Ducharme, PhD
Clinical Professor of Rehabilitation Medicine
Assistant Professor of Urology
Boston University School of Medicine

Mary Glover, MS, RNC
Director
Boston's Community Medical Group

Anantha Kamath, MD
Senior Resident in Rehabilitation Medicine

Mark Kaplan, MD
Assistant Professor of Rehabilitation Medicine
Boston University School of Medicine

Allan R. Meyers, PhD
Research Professor of Rehabilitation Medicine
Boston University School of Medicine
Professor of Health Services
Boston University School of Public Health

Jim McCormack
President
Seaside Associates

Shanker Nesathurai, MD, FRCP(C)
Assistant Professor of Rehabilitation Medicine
Boston University School of Medicine

Elizabeth Roaf, MD
Assistant Professor of Rehabilitation Medicine
Assistant Clinical Professor of Medicine
Boston University School of Medicine

John Sledge, MD
Assistant Professor of Orthopedic Surgery
Boston University School of Medicine

Jane Wierbicky, RN, BSN
Health Services Coordinator

Rehabilitation Institute of Chicago

Steven Nussbaum, MD
Assistant Professor of Rehabilitation Medicine
Northwestern University Medical School

Rehabilitation Institute of Michigan

Nancy DeSantis, DO
Assistant Professor of Rehabilitation Medicine
Wayne State University Medical School

Rancho Los Amigos Hospital

Douglas Garland, MD
Clinical Professor of Surgery
University of Southern California

Spain Rehabilitation Center

J. Scott Richards, PhD
Professor of Physical Medicine and Rehabilitation
University of Alabama at Birmingham School of Medicine

Physical Medicine Associates

Andrew Gwardjan, MD, FRCP(C)
Private Practice
Hamilton, Ontario, Canada

Chapter 1

The Epidemiology of Traumatic Spinal Cord Injury in the United States

Allan R. Meyers, PhD

Introduction

For all of the concerns about the enduring medical, social, psychological and financial consequences of SCI , little is known about the epidemiology. Moreover, much of the epidemiologic knowledge is derived from local, regional or single-state studies that are as much as 30 years old. In some notable cases, the studies are inconsistent with one another. The available studies rely upon a variety of different research methods, including hospital discharge summaries, state registries, and specialized data bases such as those maintained by the Department of Veterans Affairs (VA) and the National Model Spinal Cord Injury System (NMS). Even the most comprehensive data bases may not be representative of all people with SCI. For example, the NMS data base, estimated to include as many as 15 percent of all prevalent SCI and the source of most systematic studies of SCI epidemiology (and, not incidentally, most of the data in this chapter), is plagued by high levels of missing data on some of the most epidemiologically vital aspects of SCI. Moreover, the NMS data base is limited to adults who survive SCI, consent to inclusion in the data base, and receive treatment at an NMS center; most participating institutions are academic medical centers which may manage a more severely injured SCI population.

There have been significant improvements in the collection and analysis of SCI data. Public and private agencies, such as the Centers for Disease Control and Prevention (CDC), the U.S. Department of Education's National Institute on Disability and Rehabilitation Research (NIDRR), and the Paralyzed Veterans of America (PVA), have provided funding for some extremely interesting and useful research. For example, the CDC has sponsored the development and implementation of a number of state SCI registries. The VA has established, but not fully implemented, a national registry of spinal cord dysfunction that includes traumatic SCI. At the same time, none of our national data programs systematically report or record SCI, nor are they likely to do so in the foreseeable future. State registries have had limited success recording and tracking those injured. Despite the growing corpus of research and number of investigators, there continue to be basic questions about the epidemiology of SCI which have not been definitively answered.

Incidence, Prevalence, and Survival

With these caveats noted, the annual incidence rate appears to be about 30 to 40 new injuries per million population per year, although some local and regional studies suggest rates as high as 60 per million population per year. These figures refer only to survivors. Although there has been a trend toward improved survival and increased longevity for people with traumatic SCI, the data suggests that there are about 10 to 20 fatal injuries per million population per year; that is, injuries resulting either in immediate death or death before hospital admission. There is considerable evidence for changes in cause-specific incidence rates, but little evidence that overall incidence rates have changed in the past 30 years.

The best estimate of a prevalence rate (total number of people with SCI, in 1980) is about 700 to 900 per million population. Applying this rate to the current U.S. population suggests that there are about a quarter-million people with SCI. There is considerable evidence that acute and long-term survival has increased due to improved healthcare services and assistive technologies. Persons with SCI are living many decades after their initial injuries and now suffer from many of the same diseases that afflict individuals without SCI (i.e., cardiovascular disease, stroke, diabetes, cancer, etc.). Further advances in treatment may also decrease mortality in the SCI population and further increase the prevalence rate.

Characteristics of Injuries

The NMS data base contains the largest and most consistent data on the neurological and anatomical characteristics of SCI, with measurements at the time of initial (emergency) admission, initiation of acute rehabilitation, and rehabilitation discharge. Their data suggest that, at discharge, the most prevalent neurological levels are C5 (16 percent), C4 (13 percent), C6 (13 percent), T12 (8 percent), C7 (6 percent), and L1 (5 percent). DeVivo et. al. assert, "Overall, 52.9 percent of persons enrolled in the National SCI data base are classified as having tetraplegia (for NMS purposes, any cervical-level lesion), while 46.2 percent are classified as having paraplegia. The remaining 0.9 percent experience complete, or at least substantial, neurologic recovery by the time of discharge."

Some state and local SCI registries and other data sources show somewhat different prevalence rates, generally with higher rates of lower-level lesions. This variation may be secondary to local cultural or behavioral patterns (e.g., higher frequencies of gunshot wounds in southern and southwestern states). An alternate explanation may be that people with lower-level lesions are less likely to receive treatment in academic centers and, therefore, are less likely to be enrolled in the NMS data base.

The NMS data also suggest a trend toward more paraplegia and less tetraplegia, most notably during the decade 1981-1992. As noted below, this trend coincides with an increase in the proportion of SCI attributable to gunshots and a decrease in those related to sports. Noting the changing definitions of complete and incomplete injuries, the NMS data base reports that 52 percent of injuries are complete and 48 percent are incomplete.

Comorbid Injuries

For obvious reasons, SCI are catastrophic outcomes in their own right. Nevertheless, many people with SCI (55 percent of those in the NMS data base) experience comorbid injuries whose consequences and secondary conditions may be as clinically, psychologically and socially significant as SCI. Among these, the most prominent recorded in the NMS data base are fractures (sites unspecified; 29 percent of all SCI), head injury (12 percent; although an additional 28 percent report "loss of consciousness"), and pneumothorax or hemothorax (18 percent).

Demographics: Age, Gender, Marital Status, Ethnicity, Education, Employment, and Race

Though there may be important age-related reporting biases affecting both children and older adults, those at highest risk of SCI appear to be young adult males. There are no age-specific incidence rates. It seems prudent, however, to conclude, as DeVivo et. al. have, that "SCI occurs most frequently in teenage persons and young adults between 16 and 30 years of age." Of those enrolled in the NMS data base, the mean age at injury is about 31 years; the median age is somewhat lower at 26 years, and the mode (the age at which the greatest number of injuries took place), lower still at 19. Children (15 years or younger) account for only 4.5 percent of cases; and older adults (those 75 years of age and older), only about 1 percent. As noted, these data should be interpreted with caution. At one age extreme, the NMS does not systematically enroll children (who cannot give independent informed consent) and, therefore, may be under-represented. At the opposite extreme, the under-representation of older adults may reflect differences in incidence, survival or both. As the population ages, the numbers of older adults with SCI should increase, even if there is no change in survival.

The association with gender is clear; more than 80 percent of those enrolled in the NMS data base are males. Other data bases confirm that males are more likely to suffer from SCI [1]. There also is a close association between risk of SCI and a number of indicators of social class, all of which have profound implications for rehabilitation. For example, individuals with SCI have fewer years of education than their uninjured counterparts. They also are more likely than their uninjured counterparts to have been unemployed and to have been single (i.e., never married, separated or divorced).

Black and Hispanic men appear to be at higher risk. The NMS data base suggests that SCI affects a disproportionate number of black people; 20 percent of injuries are to blacks, although blacks constitute 12 percent of the population. As many of the NMS centers are located in inner cities, they may serve a disproportionate number of black persons. Some local and state studies suggest that Hispanic persons may have a higher risk of SCI. As the NMS data base did not begin to record data on language until 1995, the relationship among SCI, language and ethnicity is unclear; within a few years, however, there may be sufficient experience to provide more definitive data.

Cause of Injury

The largest single cause of SCI is motor vehicle collisions (MVC)[2]. MVC account for 45 percent of the cases in the NMS data base; of these, 80 percent involve automobiles[3]. Motorcycles account for another 13 percent of SCI associated with MVC (6 percent of all SCI). However, as there are substantially fewer motorcyclists than automobile drivers, the relative risk of motorcyclists experiencing SCI is very high.

In the NMS database, other common causes of SCI include falls (18 percent), intentional violence (17 percent), and sports-related injuries (13 percent). Of acts of violence, the vast majority (88 percent) are gunshot wounds. Of sports-related SCI, two-thirds are the result of diving injuries.

Of the 8 percent of SCI in the residual category ("other"), nearly half are the result of injuries associated with falling objects and a fifth are the result of iatrogenic injury.

There are close relationships among injury etiology, age, gender and, perhaps, ethnicity. Although it is not possible in such a brief review to develop these concepts in adequate detail, younger males, in general, are more likely to experience sports-related injuries, and lower-income minority males are more likely to experience injuries related to violence.

Time of Injury: Season, Day and Hour

Consistent with the premise that injuries are not accidents, SCI appear to be clustered by season, day of the week, and time of day. Though seasonal trends tend to be less noteworthy in regions of the country characterized by less temperature fluctuation, there is a clear summer peak, with the highest incidence in July. There also is a strong tendency for SCI to occur at night and on weekends: 20 percent of all SCI in the NMS data base occur on Saturday nights. These trends are most notable for injuries that are associated with motor vehicle collisions and sports.

Alcohol, Drugs and SCI

Though there is substantial evidence of the roles of alcohol use and the use of other drugs (both legal and illegal) in trauma-related mortality and morbidity, there is little specific information about their effects on the incidence of SCI. Moreover, drug and substance screening are not completed routinely and consistently in emergency departments. In addition, the biochemical markers of many cognitively clouding compounds (i.e., alcohol) are highly transitory. As such, causal connections between SCI and substance consumption are very difficult to establish.

Other Risk-Factors: Psychology, Speed and Protective Equipment

As in the cases of alcohol and drug use, it is reasonable to infer that such factors as speed (in recreational, occupational and motor vehicle settings) and the use of safety equipment (i.e., seat belts and helmets) may affect the epidemiology of SCI. In addition, psychological traits, such as "locus-of-control"[4] and "risk-taking", may affect the incidence of spinal cord injuries. However, there is little scientific evidence documenting such associations. It has been clearly demonstrated that mandatory seat belt and helmet statutes, in addition to vigorous enforcement of speeding and drunk driving laws, have reduced overall mortality. Efficacy of these interventions in reducing SCI, however, has not been studied. Increased survival of acute SCI, even when associated with a decreased incidence of MVC, may result in increased overall prevalence of SCI.

Conclusion

The three classic components of the epidemiologic triad are agent, vector and host. The characteristics of the hosts (the people who survive SCI) are most understood. Much less is known about the factors of agency and vector: matters related to protective (or destructive) equipment; social contexts of drinking, driving, work and leisure; and facility design. Knowledge about the demographic characteristics (i.e., age, gender, race) of the hosts is most complete. However, most of these factors are not amenable to intervention. The least is known about host characteristics (i.e., risk-taking behavior, excessive speed, use of protective equipment) that may be influenced by public policy initiatives. If our goal is an epidemiology that serves the purposes of prevention, as opposed to description or prediction, then new questions must be asked, and better data must be collected. Toward that goal, informed and sensitive clinicians have a critical role.

Epidemiology of Spinal Cord Injury

Incidence:	30 to 60 per million
Prevalence:	700 to 900 per million
Males to Females:	80:20
Mean Age:	31
Median Age:	26
Tetraplegia to Paraplegia:	53 percent vs. 47 percent

Blacks and Hispanics are disproportionately represented
Injuries are more likely in summer, on weekends, and at night

Etiology

Motor Vehicle Collisions	45 percent
Falls	18 percent
Violence	17 percent
Sports	13 percent
Other	8 percent

Suggested Readings

Baker, SP, O'Neill B, Karpf, editors. The injury fact book. Lexington, MA: Lexington Books, 1984.

Bracken MB, Freeman DH, Hellenbrand, K. Incidence of acute traumatic hospitalized spinal cord injury in the United States. American Journal of Epidemiology, 1981; 113:615-622.

Go BK, DeVivo MJ, Richard JS. The epidemiology of spinal cord injury. In: Stover SL, DeLisa JA, Whiteneck GG, editors. Spinal cord injury: clinical outcomes for the model systems. Gaithersburg, MD: Aspen; 1995; 21-55.

Kalsbeek WD, McLaurin RL, Harris BSH, Miller JD. The national head and spinal cord injury survey: major findings. Journal of Neurosurgery 1980: 53 (supplement); S19-S31.

Footnotes

1. For obvious reasons, VA data are virtually all male.

2. Injury epidemiologists avoid the word "accident," because it implies a random event. The preferred terms are "crashes" or "collisions." Whatever they are called, we know that such events are systematic and predictable.

3. These injuries affect drivers and passengers only. Another 2 percent of SCI affect pedestrians.

4. Locus-of-control refers to beliefs about the ability to affect personal destiny. Those with internal locus-of-control believe that they are able to affect their own destinies, including but not limited to risk of catastrophic injury; those with external locus-of-control are more fatalistic, believing that such outcomes are beyond their control.

Chapter 2

Pathophysiology of Traumatic Spinal Cord Injury

Jane Wierbicky, RN, BSN
Anantha Kamath, MD

Anatomy

The spinal cord is a complex organized mass of nerve tissues that extends distally from the level of the occiput to approximately the L2 vertebra. It is located within the vertebral canal and surrounded by the meninges.

A cross-sectional view of cord tissue reveals the butterfly-shaped gray matter surrounded by white matter. The gray matter is symmetrical and comprised of anterior, lateral and posterior horns. The gray matter is principally composed of neuronal cell bodies, but also includes dendrites, axons and glial cells (e.g., oligodendrocytes, astrocytes, etc.). The anterior horn is comprised of the cell bodies of the motor neurons. The cell bodies of the preganglionic neurons of the sympathetic nervous system are located in the lateral horn. The cell bodies of sensory fibers, which are located in the dorsal root ganglion, project into the posterior horn.

The white matter is composed of longitudinal nerve fiber tracts amid a network of neuroglia. These fibers are either myelinated or nonmyelinated and allow communication between the spinal cord and the brain. The anterior, lateral and posterior columns of the white matter each contain ascending and descending tracts.

Each of the 31 pairs of spinal nerves contain thousands of nerve fibers that branch out from the spinal cord. Each spinal nerve is composed of a dorsal and a ventral root that unite in the vicinity of the intervertebral foramen. The dorsal root conveys sensory input to the cord, and the ventral root conveys motor impulses to the skeletal muscles. The ventral root also contains efferent visceral fibers, which conduct impulses to the involuntary smooth muscles and glands of the autonomic nervous system.

Mechanism of Injury

Traumatic, nonpenetrating injury to the spinal cord generally occurs by one, or a combination, of the following mechanisms: flexion, extension, rotation or vertical compression. These actions create an external force causing the displacement of the vertebral column and consequent compression of the cord parenchyma. This traumatic event may result in vertebral fracture and/or dislocation, injury to vascular components, or ligamentous disruption or rupture. The damage to the spinal cord parenchyma is classified as concussion, contusion or laceration (including transection).

A concussion is characterized by transient neurological symptoms with rapid resolution of deficits. No notable gross anatomic lesions are identifiable. As well, true cord concussion is rarely seen.

Cord contusion is frequently encountered in traumatic SCI. Classically, it is the result of the compression of the spinal cord. Although the gross structural continuity of the cord remains intact, the cord is bruised in appearance. This is a result of petechial hemorrhage into surrounding tissues.

Cord lacerations are the result of severe displacements of the vertebral column. The bony fragments of vertebral fractures may retropulse into the spinal canal and thereby cause grossly visible laceration or disruption of the cord tissues. Traumatic intervertebral disc herniations could impinge upon the spinal cord and associated vasculature. Membranes may be torn and, in some instances, the cord may be completely transected. Due to the ensuing damage to the motor, sensory and autonomic pathways, there may be partial or complete loss of function below the level of the lesion.

Missile Injuries to the Spinal Cord

The extent of tissue injury sustained from a missile wound is directly related to the mass and velocity of the projectile. As a bullet passes through tissue, a wound track is formed. The structures that are immediately adjacent to this track (i.e., bone and ligaments) are displaced with such speed and force that they themselves act as secondary missiles. Bullets may fragment and ricochet, which can increase the amount of neurological injury. Retained missile fragments may cause a foreign body reaction in the spinal cord. In addition, there is a high incidence of infection. Antibiotics and tetanus toxoid should be considered.

Progression of Lesion Development in Moderate and Severe SCI

A secondary chain of cellular events is set into motion immediately following the initial insult to the spinal cord. The pathophysiology of the injury can be divided into three stages: acute, intermediate and late.

Acute Stage

Inflammatory reactions (i.e., edema, hyperemia, hemorrhage) of the spinal cord may develop immediately post-injury. The cell membranes are highly permeable in the acute stage, and edema may be present up to 15 days post-injury. The endothelial cells of the intact capillaries become edematous, thereby limiting perfusion and resulting in ischemia. There may be further risk of ischemic damage in persons experiencing hypovolemic shock or those requiring cardiopulmonary resuscitation. Damage to the spinal vasculature and thrombosis may also result in further ischemia.

Monocytes are mobilized from the damaged vessels and are eventually converted to macrophages. The macrophages will begin their phagocytic role in the gray matter of the cord and remove necrotic debris from the area of injury. This process of phagocytosis will continue until the debris is removed and a central cavity develops. Nerve compromise is manifested by traumatic demyelination and fragmentation changes of the axonal cylinders. Vacuoles may develop in the white matter secondary to the breakdown of the myelin sheaths surrounding the axons. After several days, glial cells proliferate, forming astrocytic fibers between the necrotic cavity and the intact tissue. These cavities, which represent sites of complete parenchymal hemorrhagic necrosis, may be singular or multilocular.

Intermediate Stage

After several weeks, the cavity is fully developed and gliosis is complete. The edema has resolved and the cord appears atrophied. The meninges have become fibrotic, and the subarachnoid space at the level of the injury is sometimes obliterated.

Anterior and posterior nerve root regeneration becomes apparent.

Late Stage

Several months post-injury, the cyst wall is thick. Collagenous fibrosis is present in varying degrees and is generally proportional to the degree of initial hemorrhage. Arachnoiditis may develop due to scarring of the membranes. In many cases, there is a degree of preserved white matter at the periphery of the lesion. Nerve root regeneration is present in most cases within one year post-injury.

Numerous complications may be encountered several years post-injury. Post-traumatic syringomyelia develops in 5 percent of the SCI population. Although the exact mechanism is unclear, chronic mechanical stress to the spinal cord (i.e., kyphosis, canal stenosis) may contribute to the development of a syrinx (see chapter 16). This post-traumatic cyst may progressively ascend or descend over many segments of the spinal cord. There may be a decrease in neurological function noted, and surgery to drain the cyst may be warranted. Osteoarthritis may also lead to further neurological decline. Osteophytes and herniated disks may impinge upon the spinal cord vasculature, impairing blood flow and resulting in ischemic changes. Traumatic neuromas arising from the spinal nerve roots are also occasionally encountered.

Conclusion

The pathophysiology of traumatic spinal cord injury is complex and cannot be fully summarized in this brief review. In addition, many biological aspects of SCI warrant further investigation. An understanding of the concepts, however, provides a useful foundation for clinical practice.

Suggested Readings

Abel R, Gerner HJ, Smit C, Meiners T. Residual deformity of the spinal canal in patients with traumatic paraplegia and secondary changes of the spinal cord. Spinal Cord 1999; 37:14-19.

Kakulas BA, Taylor J. Pathophysiology of injuries of the vertebral column and spinal cord. In: Vinken PJ, editor. Handbook of clinical neurology: spinal cord trauma (vol. 17). New York: Elsevier Science Publishers, 1992.

Kakulas BA. The applied neuropathology of human spinal cord injury. Spinal Cord 1999; 37:79-88.

Noback C, Demarest R. The nervous system: introduction and review. New York: McGraw-Hill, 1972.

Yashon D. Spinal injury. New York: Appleton-Century-Crofts, 1978.

Chapter 3

Surgical Management of Spine Fractures

John Sledge, MD
Dain Allred

In the United States, spinal cord injuries are usually treated in tertiary care centers. Proper acute management requires the skills of a trauma team that is composed of nurses, emergency room physicians, general surgeons, orthopedic surgeons, neurological surgeons, and anesthesiologists. Rehabilitation clinicians, although not intimately involved with the emergent management, must have a basic understanding of the acute issues.

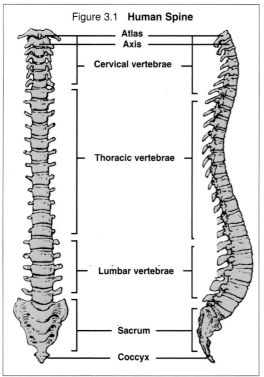

Figure 3.1 **Human Spine**

Atlas
Axis
Cervical vertebrae
Thoracic vertebrae
Lumbar vertebrae
Sacrum
Coccyx

Anatomy

The spine has seven cervical vertebrae, 12 thoracic vertebrae, five lumbar vertebrae, and five sacral vertebrae (Figures 3.1, 3.2 and 3.3). The sacral vertebrae are fused. The spine provides strong protection for the spinal cord except in the most violent of traumatic events. The terminal portion of the spinal cord is the conus medularis, which becomes the cauda equina ("horse's tail") at approximately the L2 vertebral level.

Clinical Evaluation

When a patient is involved in a significant trauma, an SCI should be suspected. At a minimum, a thorough clinical examination must be completed and lateral cervical spine X-ray must be ordered. Approximately 5 percent of patients with a spine injury will have a noncontiguous second lesion. If SCI cannot be excluded with standard films, then further investigations, in-

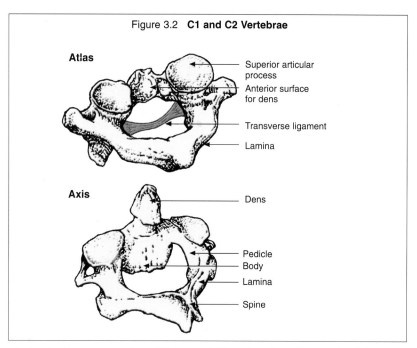

Figure 3.2 **C1 and C2 Vertebrae**

Atlas
- Superior articular process
- Anterior surface for dens
- Transverse ligament
- Lamina

Axis
- Dens
- Pedicle
- Body
- Lamina
- Spine

cluding flexion-extension views, CT scans or MRI studies, should be completed. Unrecognized SCI can result in devastating clinical and medicolegal consequences.

The spine surgeon is concerned with the following issues. First, has the patient been appropriately resuscitated and stabilized (i.e., airway, breathing, circulation)? Second, is there a spinal injury and, if so, what type of injury is present? Third, does the patient have any neurological deficit secondary to spinal cord compromise (i.e., contusion, transection)? Fourth, on the basis of clinical examination, injury pattern and radiological studies, is the injury stable or unstable? Finally, is the treatment operative or non-operative (i.e., collar, SOMI brace, halo)? If the injury is unstable or there is neurological compromise, surgical intervention should be considered. The nature of the injury will determine whether operative intervention will be from an anterior or posterior approach, or both. The type of injury will also dictate if operative treatment involves decompression, instrumentation and/or fusion. The timing of surgery in an unstable injury with neurological deficits is somewhat controversial. Some would argue that surgery should be delayed until spinal cord edema has diminished; others believe delay in definitive treatment is unnecessary. Although treatment must be individualized, the following are some general guidelines for surgical management.

Methylprednisolone

The National Acute Spinal Cord Injury 2 (NASCIS 2) study randomized non-penetrating acute SCI patients to placebo, high dose methylprednisolone or naloxone. Patients with exclusively cauda equina lesions (i.e., L3 burst fracture) and penetrating wounds (i.e., gunshot injuries, stabbings) were excluded. Patients were enrolled within 12 hours of injury. Those assigned to the steroid arm received a bolus of 30 mg/kg, with a continuous infusion of 5.4 mg/kg/hr for 23 hours. Overall, there was no difference among the three treatment arms. There was, however, a reported benefit among those patients treated within eight hours of injury.

NASCIS 3 randomized patients to 24 hours of steroids, 48 hours of steroids, or tirilazad mesylate. Again, there was no significant difference among the three treatment arms when all of the patients are considered. However, 48 hours of methylprednisolone was reported to benefit those patients treated within three to eight hours of injury.

The statistical analysis and clinical significance of the putative gains attributed to methylprednisolone in both of these studies are not universally accepted. However, treatment with methlyprednisolone is commonly accepted practice in Canada and the United States.

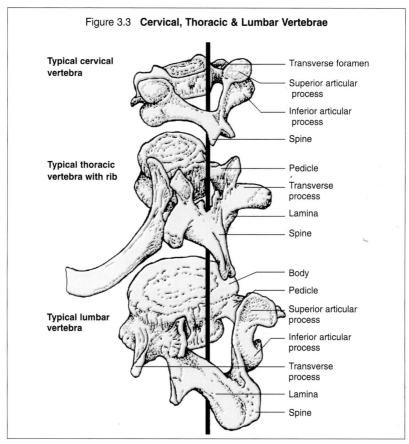

Figure 3.3 **Cervical, Thoracic & Lumbar Vertebrae**

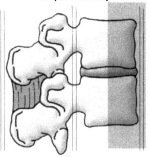

Figure 3.4 **Three Column Model of Spine Stability**

Anterior Column

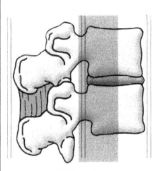

Middle Column

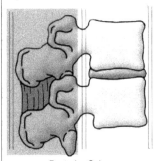

Posterior Column

Spine Stability

In general, the stability of fractures of the occipital condyle, axis (C1) and atlas (C2) are determined by fracture pattern. Spinal stability of fractures of the lower cervical spine (C3 to C7) can be assessed by the criterion described by White and Punjabi. This system requires assessment of translation and angulation in cervical flexion and extension films. In general, relative sagittal plane translation of 3.5 mm is associated with instability. Likewise, relative sagittal plane angulation of greater than 11 degrees is associated with instability.

The stability of thoracic and lumbar injuries is evaluated by utilizing the three-column model described by Denis (Figure 3.4). The anterior column consists of the anterior longitudinal ligament, anterior vertebral body, and anterior annulus fibrosis. The middle column consists of the posterior vertebral body, posterior annulus fibrosis, posterior longitudinal ligament and spinal cord. The posterior column includes the spinous process, laminae, facets, pedicles and posterior ligamentous structures (i.e., ligamentum flavum, intraspinous ligaments, supraspinous ligaments). Fractures are deemed stable if there is compromise to only one column. The spine is considered unstable when two or more columns are compromised.

Cervical Spine Injuries

Occipital Condyle Injuries

Occipital condyle injuries are rare and can be classified into three different groups. Type 1 injuries are impaction injuries secondary to axial loading. Type 2 injuries are associated with basal skull fractures. Type 1 and Type 2 fractures are stable and can be treated with a cervical orthosis (i.e., Philadelphia collar, SOMI brace). Type 3 injuries are secondary to violent lateral or rotational forces and are associated with alar ligament avulsion. If there is instability, operative treatment is required.

Posterior Arch Fracture

Mechanism: combined extension and lateral loading

Treatment: stable injury; initial treatment with cervical collar or halo

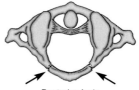

Posterior Arch

Lateral Mass Fracture

Mechanism: combined axial loading and lateral bending

Treatment: stable injury; cervical collar or halo

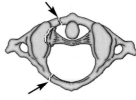

Lateral Mass

Jefferson Burst Fracture

Mechanism: axial loading causing fractures of anterior and posterior parts of the atlas

Treatment: halo if excursion of lateral masses is greater than 8 mm; otherwise hard collar; if symptomatic nonunion after three months, then occiput to C2 fusion is required

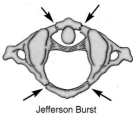

Jefferson Burst

Anterior Arch Fracture

Mechanism: combined axial load and flexion

Treatment: hard collar

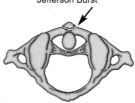

Anterior Arch

Transverse Process Fracture

Mechanism: avulsion injury

Treatment: usually an incidental finding requiring only symptomatic treatment

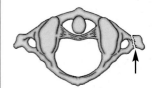

Transverse Process

Figure 3.5 **C1 (Atlas) Fractures**

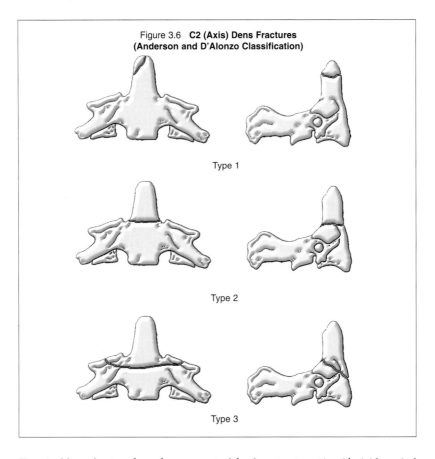

Figure 3.6 **C2 (Axis) Dens Fractures (Anderson and D'Alonzo Classification)**

Type 1

Type 2

Type 3

Type 1: oblique fracture through upper part of the dens; treatment is with rigid cervical orthosis such as Philadelphia collar

Type 2: fracture at the junction of the odontoid process and the vertebral body; if displacement is less than 5 mm and angulated less than 15 degrees, then halo is appropriate; otherwise operative treatment with C1 to C2 fusion or screw fixation

Type 3: fracture extends down through vertebral body; treatment is with halo

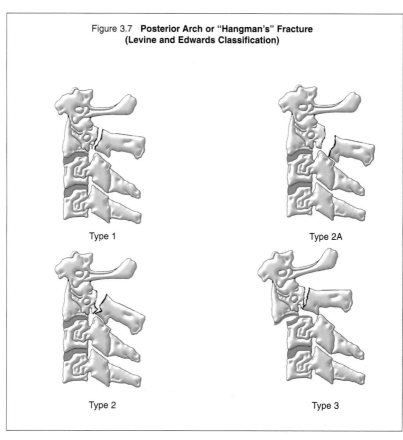

Figure 3.7 **Posterior Arch or "Hangman's" Fracture (Levine and Edwards Classification)**

Type 1

Type 2A

Type 2

Type 3

Type 1: fracture with no angulation and less than 3 mm of translation; treatment is with halo

Type 2: fracture with significant angulation and translation (>3 mm); treatment is with halo after closed reduction

Type 2A: fracture with severe angulation but with minimal anterior translation; fragments appear to hinge on the anterior longitudinal ligament; treatment is with halo after closed reduction

Type 3: fracture-dislocation with severe angulation and translation with unilateral or bilateral facet dislocation; treatment is with C1 to C2 fusion

Injuries of the Lower Cervical Spine

There is no clearly accepted classification system. As such, a descriptive system is employed. The basic principles of fracture management apply (i.e., treatment-based stability and presence of neurological deficit).

Spinous Process Fracture (Clay-Shoveler's Fracture)
   Mechanism: flexion injury with avulsion of spinous process; this is a stable injury
   Treatment: requires only symptomatic treatment

Extension Avulsion (Teardrop Fracture)
   Mechanism: hyperextension avulsion of the antero-inferior vertebral body
   Treatment: hard collar

Lamina or Lateral Mass Fracture
   Mechanism: posterior element fracture most often from compressive-extension
   Treatment: hard collar

Facet Dislocation (Unilateral or Bilateral)
   Mechanism: inferior and superior facets are not fractured, however, the superior articular process is anterior to the inferior articular process; this is a flexion distraction injury
   Treatment: if patient is awake, then emergent closed reduction; if patient is not awake, then MRI prior to closed reduction to rule out associated disk herniation; if closed reduction is unsuccessful, then open reduction is necessary

Facet Fracture (Unilateral or Bilateral)
   Mechanism: one of the two articular processes is fractured, with or without a change in the relationship of the inferior to superior facet; this is a flexion compression injury
   Treatment: if patient is awake, then emergent closed reduction; many times, closed reduction is unsuccessful, and open reduction is necessary

Flexion Teardrop
   Mechanism: fracture of the anterior vertebral body from a flexion compression injury
   Treatment: anterior decompression and fusion

Compression Fracture
   Mechanism: axial load injury
   Treatment: hard collar or halo if no instability or malalignment; otherwise anterior interbody fusion

Burst Fracture
   Mechanism: comminuted fracture of vertebral body fracture secondary to axial loading
   Treatment: hard collar or halo if no instability or malalignment; otherwise anterior interbody fusion; if neurologic injury, then anterior decompression prior to fusion

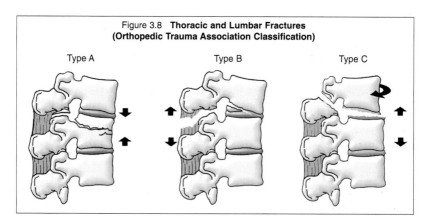

Figure 3.8 **Thoracic and Lumbar Fractures (Orthopedic Trauma Association Classification)**

Type A - Vertebral Body Compression
Mechanism: most common injuries caused by axial compression with or without flexion; vertebral body height reduced, but posterior ligamentous complex is intact

Treatment: if stable and no neurological deficit, then brace for three months; if neurological deficit, spine instability or significant deformity is present, then decompression and fusion

Type B - Anterior and Posterior Element Injury with Distraction
Mechanism: fracture with disruption of one or more columns; flexion initiates posterior disruption and elongation, while hyperextension causes anterior disruption and elongation; three subtypes

Treatment: if stable and no neurological deficit, then brace for three months; if neurological deficit is present or spine is unstable, then decompression and fusion

Type C - Anterior and Posterior Element Injury with Rotation
Mechanism: most severe injuries, associated with highest rate of neurological deficit; disruption of all longitudinal ligaments, disks, and articular process fracture; three subtypes
Treatment: fusion, with or without decompression.

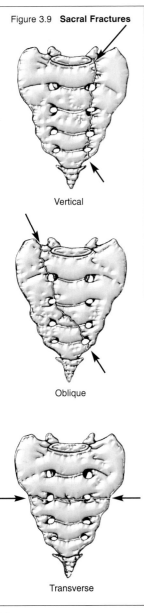

Figure 3.9 **Sacral Fractures**

Vertical

Oblique

Transverse

Vertical
Fracture line traverses ala, foramen or body of the sacrum

Oblique
May occur at any level and may be associated with concomitant pelvic fracture

Transverse
Least common sacral fracture, but most likely to have neurological deficit

Treatment: most sacral fractures are stable, minimally displaced, and are not associated with neurological deficits; in these cases symptomatic treatment is appropriate (i.e., rest, NSAID, etc.); those injuries associated with neurological deficit require decompression and stabilization; goals of operative management are to reestablish pelvic ring and lumbosacral junction stability, correct and/or prevent angulation or displacement, and prevent neurologic deterioration.

Suggested Readings

Anderson L, D'Alonzo R. Fractures of the odontoid process of the axis. Journal of Bone Joint Surgery 1974; 56A:663-674.

Bracken MB, Shepard MJ, Collins WF, et. al. A randomized controlled trial of methylprednisolone or naloxone in the treatment of acute spinal cord injury. New England Journal of Medicine 1990; 322:1405-1411.

Bracken, MB, Shepard MJ, Holford TR, et. al. Administration of methylprednisolone for 24 or 48 hours or tirilazad mesylate for 48 hours in the treatment of acute spinal cord injury. Journal of the American Medical Association 1997: 277:1597-1604.

Denis F. The three column spine and its significance in the classification of acute thoracolumbar spine injuries. Spine 1983; 8:817-831.

Levin A, Edwards C. Treatment of injuries in the C1-C2 complex. Orthop Clin North Am 1986; 17:31-44.

Magerl F, Aebi M, Gertzbein S, Harms J, Nazarian S. A comprehensive classification of the thoracic and lumbar injuries. European Spine Journal 1994; 3:184-201.

Nesathurai S. Steroids and spinal cord injury: Revisiting NASCIS 2 and NASCIS 3 trials. Journal of Trauma 1998; 45:1088-1093.

White A, Southwick W, Punjabi M. Clinical instability in the lower cervical spine: A review of past and current concepts. Spine 1976; 1:15.

Chapter 4

Clinical and Functional Evaluation

Shanker Nesathurai, MD, FRCP(C)
Andrew Gwardjan, MD, FRCP(C)

Clinicians must incorporate the rehabilitation paradigm into their clinical practice. As such, physiatrists must understand the functional consequences of a medical condition. In other words, how does a disorder prevent a patient from performing important life tasks? The activities of daily living (ADL) are the elementary tasks that must be completed for a patient to achieve a basic quality of life. These tasks include dressing, bathing, toileting, feeding, grooming, transfers, ambulating and communicating. The instrumental activities of daily living (IADL) are those essential tasks that allow individuals to interact with the broader community. These tasks include grocery shopping, banking and laundry. Clearly, there is no distinct demarcation between ADL and IADL. These ADL and IADL can be performed independently, with modified independence (i.e., with a device), with supervision, or with the assistance of one or even two caregivers.

Once ADL and IADL goals have been reached, patients may pursue vocational and avocational goals. Vocational pursuits may range from unpaid volunteer work (i.e., therapeutic employment) to working with adaptive devices (modified work) to competitive employment. Avocational pursuits include hobbies and recreational activities such as playing chess and water skiing.

Pyramid of Function

Avocational Activities
Vocational Activities
Instrumental Activities of Daily Living
Activities of Daily Living

Levels of Independence

Independent
Modified independence with technology and/or assistive devices
Supervised independence
Assistance of one person
Assistance of two persons

World Health Organization Definition of Impairment, Disability and Handicap

Impairment is the lack of normal anatomical or psychological function. Disability is, as the result of an impairment, the inability to perform functional tasks. Handicap is the social disadvantage secondary to a disability. For example, an impairment would be a fractured humerus. As the result of this impairment, the individual requires assistance in certain activities of daily living (ADL), such as dressing and grooming. This individual's handicap is partly determined by his premorbid social, financial and vocational status. If he were a psychiatrist who could walk to work, he would have essentially no handicap. On the other hand, if he were a neurosurgeon, he would be unable to work, and thus would be significantly handicapped.

A number of instruments to measure function have been developed, such as the Functional Independence Measure (FIM), Barthel Index, Sister Kenny Index, and Quadriplegia Index of Function. The FIM is the most widely used functional instrument for general rehabilitation units in North America. However, this instrument may not be sensitive or appropriate for functional assessment in SCI patients.

Physicians and surgeons are adept at identifying and treating impairments. Therapists are skilled at optimizing functional capabilities. Physiatrists must identify impairments, but also understand the resulting functional limitations. Rehabilitation physicians must coordinate the treatment plans of the entire health-care team to optimize clinical outcomes.

Evaluating SCI Patients

Every SCI patient should be thoroughly evaluated by a physician. This clinical assessment includes a complete physical examination. The American Spinal Injury Association (ASIA) scoring system is the most commonly accepted impairment evaluation paradigm. This system (Table 3) classifies patients on the basis of their clinical exam, and not by radiological or anatomical abnormalities. The essential elements include the bilateral assessment of 10 index muscles (Table 1) and 28 dermatomes. Rectal sensation and voluntary sphincteric contraction are also evaluated. In addition to the elements of the ASIA examination, a general medical examination, including mental status, cranial nerves and reflexes, should be completed.

The index muscles are assessed in the supine position. Each index muscle receives a score from 0 to 5 (Table 2). The motor level is the lowest index muscle with at least 3 grade strength; all cephalad muscles must have 5 grade strength. Thus, a left and right motor level can be obtained. The motor level is deemed the most caudal segment with normal motor function. The "final" motor level is the higher of the left and right motor levels. The motor score is the sum of the individual motor assessment from each index muscle. This value ranges from 0 to 100.

Table 1
Key ASIA Muscles That Must Be Examined

Myotomes	Index Muscle	Action
C5	Biceps, Brachialis	Elbow flexors
C6	Extensor Carpi Radialis	Wrist extensors
C7	Triceps	Elbow extensors
C8	Flexor Digitorum Profundus	Finger flexors
T1	Abductor Digiti Minimi	Small finger abductors
L2	Iliopsoas	Hip flexors
L3	Quadriceps	Knee extensors
L4	Tibialis Anterior	Ankle dorsiflexors
L5	Extensor Halicus Longus	Long toe extensors
S1	Gastrocnemius	Ankle plantarflexors

Table 2
Assessment of Strength

0	Total paralysis
1	Palpable or visible contraction
2	Active movement, full range of movement with gravity eliminated
3	Active movement, full range of movement against gravity
4	Active movement, full range of movement against moderate resistance
5	Normal active movement, full range of movement against full resistance

Light touch and pinprick are assessed from 28 dermatomes bilaterally. For every segment, a score of 0 (absent), 1 (impaired), and 2 (normal) is determined for each modality. Four different scores are generated: left light touch, right light touch, left pinprick, and right pinprick. The sensory score is the sum of the dermatomal sensory scores for each modality and range from 0 to 112. Based on this clinical assessment, a sensory level can be determined for the left and right sides of the body. The sensory level is defined as the highest level with entirely normal sensory function (i.e., both pinprick and light touch). The "final" sensory level is the higher of the left and right sensory levels.

The rectal exam is an essential element of the ASIA scoring system. The examiner's finger must be placed in the rectum, and the patient must be asked if he perceives any sensation. The patient is also asked to "bear down" on the examiner's finger to determine if volitional contraction of the sphincter exists.

The neurological level is the most caudal spinal segment with entirely normal function. Evaluation of the C5 to T1 and L4 to S1 segments involves the assessment of a motor and sensory function. However, all other segments (C2 to C4, T2 to T12 and S2 to S4/5) require only an assessment of sensory function. To determine the neurological level, it is helpful to review the left and right motor and sensory levels. For example, a patient with a left and right C7 motor level and a left and right C6 sensory level would be assigned a C6 neurological level. However, motor function in the thoracic spinal segments below the T1 level are not scored with the ASIA paradigm. Sensation (pinprick and light touch) is the only function that is scored between the T2 and T12 segments. Consider the case where an individual had a 5 grade power in all the index muscles of the upper extremity (i.e., left and right T1 motor level) and 0 grade power in the lower extremities. In addition, this person had a left and right T8 sensory level. In this example, the neurological level assigned would be T8.

In summary, four different levels are obtained: left motor, right motor, left sensory and right sensory. On occasion, the process of assigning a neurological level results in misrepresentation of a patient's true impairment. This is particularly evident when there is a marked discrepancy between the motor and sensory levels, or in a lesion with asymmetrical motor and sensory findings. It is advisable to document all four levels, in addition to the final neurological level. The ASIA impairment rating provides a framework to classify injuries as complete or incomplete. To categorize an injury as incomplete, there must be some intact sensory or motor function in the S4/5 segments; this is manifested by some sensation at the anal musculocutaneous junction, deep anal sensation on rectal examination, or voluntary contraction of the anal sphincter.

The zone of partial preservation (ZPP) refers to the number of partially intact dermatomes and myotomes caudal to the neurological level. By ASIA directive, the ZPP should only be calculated in complete lesions.

Table 3
ASIA Impairment Scale

A   Complete: No sensory or motor function is preserved in the sacral segments S4/5.

B   Sensory Incomplete: Sensory but no motor function is preserved below the neurological level and includes the sacral segments S4/5.

C   Motor Incomplete: Motor function is preserved below the neurological level, and more than half of the key muscles below the neurological level have a muscle grade less than 3. There must be some sparing of sensory and/or motor function in the sacral segments S4/5.

D   Motor Incomplete: Motor function is preserved below the neurological level, and at least half of the key muscles below the neurological level have a muscle grade greater than or equal to 3. There must be some sparing of sensory and/or motor function in the sacral segments S4/5.

E   Normal: Sensory and motor function are normal. Patient may have abnormalities on reflex examination.

Steps In Assigning an ASIA Level

1. Examine 10 index muscles bilaterally
2. Examine 28 dermatomes bilaterally for pinprick and light tough
3. Complete rectal exam to assess sensation and volitional sphincteric contraction
4. Determine left and right motor levels
5. Determine left and right sensory levels
6. Assign "final" motor and sensory levels
7. Determine neurological level, which is the most caudal segment with normal motor and sensory function
8. Categorize injury as complete or incomplete by ASIA impairment scale (A, B, C, D, E)
9. Calculate motor and sensory score
10. Determine zone of partial preservation if complete injury ("A" on impairment scale)

Table 4
Reflexes and Corresponding Nerve Roots

Stretch Reflex	Predominant Motor/Root Level
Biceps	C5
Brachioradialis	C6
Triceps	C7
Finger Flexor	C8
Quadriceps	L4
Hamstrings	L5
Gastrocnemius	S1

Discrepancy Between Anatomical and ASIA Neurological Level

Many times, there is a discrepancy between the anatomical level of injury and the neurolgical level. For example, a patient with a C6 burst fracture may have sparing of the

ASIA Scoring of Hypothetical Patient with a C6C (Motor Incomplete) Injury

MOTOR

KEY MUSCLES

	R	L	
C2			
C3			
C4			
C5	5	5	Elbow flexors
C6	5	5	Wrist extensors
C7	5	2	Elbow extensors
C8	5	0	Finger flexors (distal phalanx of middle finger)
T1	4	1	Finger abductors (little finger)
T2			
T3			
T4			
T5			
T6			
T7			
T8			
T9			
T10			
T11			
T12			
L1			
L2	0	1	Hip flexors
L3	0	0	Knee extensors
L4	3	2	Ankle dorsiflexors
L5	2	2	Long toe extensors
S1	0	0	Ankle plantar flexors
S2			
S3			
S4-5			

0 = total paralysis
1 = palpable or visible contraction
2 = active movement, gravity eliminated
3 = active movement, against gravity
4 = active movement, against some resistance
5 = active movement, against full resistance
NT= not testable

Yes Voluntary anal contraction (Yes/No)

TOTALS 29 + 18 = 47 **MOTOR SCORE**

(MAXIMUM) (50) (50) (100)

SENSORY

KEY SENSORY POINTS

	LIGHT TOUCH R	LIGHT TOUCH L	PIN PRICK R	PIN PRICK L
C2	2	2	2	2
C3	2	2	2	2
C4	2	2	2	2
C5	2	2	2	2
C6	2	2	2	2
C7	2	2	2	2
C8	2	2	2	2
T1	2	2	2	2
T2	2	1	2	1
T3	2	2	2	2
T4	0	0	0	0
T5	0	0	0	0
T6	0	0	0	0
T7	0	0	0	0
T8	0	0	0	0
T9	0	0	0	0
T10	0	0	0	0
T11	0	0	0	0
T12	0	0	0	0
L1	0	0	0	0
L2	0	0	0	0
L3	0	0	0	0
L4	0	0	0	0
L5	0	0	0	0
S1	0	0	0	0
S2	0	0	0	0
S3	0	0	0	0
S4-5	2	2	2	2

0 = absent
1 = impaired
2 = normal
NT= not testable

Yes Any anal sensation (Yes/No)

TOTALS 22 + 21 = 43 **PIN PRICK SCORE** (max: 112)

22 + 21 = 43 **LIGHT TOUCH SCORE** (max: 112)

(MAXIMUM) (56) (56) (56) (56)

• Key Sensory Points

NEUROLOGICAL LEVEL
The most caudal segment with normal function

	R	L
SENSORY	T3	T1
MOTOR	T1	C6

COMPLETE OR INCOMPLETE? Incomplete
Incomplete = presence of any sensory or motor function in lowest sacral segment

ZONE OF PARTIAL PRESERVATION
Partially innervated segments

	R	L
SENSORY	NA	NA
MOTOR	NA	NA

(From International Standards for Neurological and Functional Classification of Spinal Cord Injury. Reprinted with permission of American Spinal Injury Association, Chicago, 1992.)

C7 motor level. This is because the motor neuron pool for any myotome is cephalad to the corresponding vertebral body. As a guideline, the motor neuron pool is one segment cephalad to the corresponding vertebral body in the cervical spine, two segments higher in the thoracic spine, and three segments higher in the lumbar spine.

Complete vs. Incomplete Injury

Complete injuries imply that there is not any significant function below the level of injury. The ASIA scoring system provides some standardization of the definitions; however, most patients (and some clinicians) do not characterize injuries on the basis of the most recent ASIA criterion. As such, these terms can be a source of confusion.

On rare occasions, the ASIA definition of a complete injury can be inconsistent with clinical intuition. Consider the case of an individual with a 5 grade power in the biceps (C5 myotome) and 4 grade power in the wrist extensors (C6 myotome) with 2 to 3 grade strength in the L2, L3, and L4 index muscles. Assume strength in all other index muscles are 0 grade, and rectal tone and sensation are absent. In addition, the motor exam is the same on both the left and right side. Intuitively, this patient has some strength below the level of the lesion and, arguably, should be classified as an incomplete motor injury with a C6 motor level. Under the current ASIA scoring paradigm, there must be some volitional rectal sphincter contraction and/or rectal sensation to categorize an injury as incomplete. This hypothetical patient would be classified as a C6 complete lesion. It should be noted that the ASIA paradigm does require that the zone of partial preservation (ZPP) be calculated in complete injuries. Documenting the ZPP would further clarify this patient's clinical presentation.

Upper and Lower Motor Neuron Injury

It is important to understand the concept of upper and lower motor neuron injury. Volitional movement of muscle groups requires an intact upper and lower motor neuron supply. The upper motor neuron supply (i.e., corticospinal tract) begins in the prefrontal motor cortex, travels through the internal capsule and brain stem, and projects into the spinal cord. The lower motor neuron supply begins in the anterior horn cells of the spinal cord and includes the peripheral nerves. Most lesions in the cervical and thoracic cord result in predominantly upper motor neuron injury. However, at the level of the injury, there may be limited lower motor neuron injury with compromise of the nerve roots and/or the anterior horn cells. Upper motor neuron lesions are associated with upper motor neuron findings such as increased muscle stretch reflexes, clonus, babinski (extensor) response, and detrusor sphincter dyssynergia. The terminal segment of the spinal cord, the conus medularis, is located at approximately the L1 to L2 vertebral body. Injuries below the L2 vertebral body result in lower motor neuron injury. Lower motor neuron lesions are characterized by hyporeflexia, flaccid weakness, and significant muscle wasting. Lesions at the upper lumbar vertebral bodies can present with a mixture of upper and lower motor neuron findings.

Spinal Shock

It is sometimes difficult to clinically distinguish between upper and lower motor neuron injury after SCI due to "spinal shock." Spinal shock is a commonly used term that refers to the lack of descending facilitation after an upper motor neuron lesion. The patient will initially have findings consistent with lower motor neuron injury, although upper motor neuron findings will typically develop over a period of days to weeks.

Suggested Readings

Maynard FM, Bracken MB, Creasey G, Ditunno JF, et al. International standards for neurological and functional classification of spinal cord injury. Spinal Cord 1997; 35:266-274.

Chapter 5

Functional Outcomes By Level of Injury

Shanker Nesathurai, MD, FRCP(C)

Patients, families and clinicians may inquire about an individual's ultimate functional capability after completing a rehabilitation program. Physicians must be able to provide cautious, but realistic advice. The following is a general discussion of functional capability by motor level. Although not the exclusive determinant, functional independence is closely correlated with motor level.

With the exception of a complete anatomical spinal cord transection, it is difficult to predict with confidence on the ultimate return of function distal to the neurological level. It is not unusual for individuals to gain one motor level over the first year of injury. Some patients with devastating injuries regain significant power distal to their level of injury; others make no recovery whatsoever.

C2 to C4 Tetraplegia

Patients with C2 to C4 lesions are the most profoundly injured SCI patients and are commonly referred to as "high tetraplegics." These patients have no significant strength in any limb. Many are ventilator dependent and have long-term tracheostomies. These patients require assistance for all ADL and IADL. A caregiver must be available on a 24-hour basis. Mobility requires a power wheelchair. Intermittent catheterization is ideal, but an attendant must be available to perform this procedure four to six times per day. As a practical matter, most high tetraplegics have an indwelling urinary catheter (Foley or suprapubic).

Technological advances have clearly improved the quality of these patients' lives. A ventilator dependent patient may require a "talking" tracheostomy tube to communicate. Computer-driven environmental control systems that interface with voice, sip-and-puff, or chin control mechanisms allow patients to perform tasks such as turning on lights or opening a door.

The phrenic nerve supplies the diaphragm and is supplied by the C3, C4, and C5 motor neuron pool. On occasion, "pacing" the phrenic nerve with an electrical stimulator can liberate a high tetraplegic from the ventilator for at least part of the day. However, the lower motor neuron pathways must be intact to pace the nerve. Nerve conduction studies of the phrenic nerve and an EMG of the diaphragm can help determine if pacing is a viable option.

C5 Tetraplegia

Patients with this motor level have some preserved biceps function. These individuals should be able to assist in their self-care activities (e.g., grooming, bathing and toileting). C5 tetraplegics will require adaptive devices to feed independently (e.g., universal cuffs). C5 tetraplegics cannot perform intermittent self-catheterization. As a practical matter, bladder management will require an indwelling catheter. C5 tetraplegics will require assistance for transfers. Mobility will be with a power wheelchair.

C6 Tetraplegia

Preservation of the C6 myotome confers significant functional advantages. C6 tetraplegics have intact wrist extension. This allows for the utilization of the tenodesis effect, in which the active movement of wrist extensors results in passive movement of the digits. The result is a type of prehension that will increase functional independence.

C6 tetraplegics may, with proper training, be able to achieve modified independence in dressing and bathing. In both males and females, bowel care on the commode may be performed with modified independence. Males at this level of impairment may be able to perform self-catherization. With a sliding board, transfers may be completed without the assistance of a caregiver. This is the most cephalad level at which a manual wheelchair may be used. Some individuals will be able to use a manual wheelchair for all actitivies; others will require a power wheelchair for community mobility. C6 tetraplegics may be able to drive a modified van.

C7 and C8 Tetraplegia

C7 tetraplegics have some function in the triceps muscles. With intact triceps function, transfers should be independent without a sliding board. At this level, patients should be independent in most functional tasks at a modified level. Both male and female patients should be able to perform intermittent bladder catheterization. A manual wheelchair can be used both indoors and outdoors. Some individuals at this level of injury may be able to drive a modified automobile.

Thoracic Paraplegia (T1 to T12 Neurological Level)

The intercostal muscles are innervated by the thoracic spinal cord from the T1 to T12 segments. The upper abdominal (T8 to T10) and lower abdominal muscles (T11 to T12) are also supplied by the thoracic spinal cord.

The more caudal the lesion, the greater number of intercostal muscles are spared. As such, a patient with a lower thoracic (T10) lesion will have more truncal stability in a wheelchair than a patient with a higher lesion (T2). A low thoracic paraplegic is more likely to have intact abdominal and intercostal muscles, which will improve coughing and secretion clearance. Generally, patients with lesions below the T6 level are not at risk for autonomic dysreflexia.

Thoracic paraplegics should achieve modified independent self care and transfers, as well as bowel and bladder managment. Mobility will be with a manual wheelchair. Most thoracic paraplegics should be able to drive a modified automobile.

Lumbar Paraplegia

SCI patients with some strength in the lower extremities may be able to ambulate. In addition to muscle strength, walking requires adequate sensation, coordination, joint range, and cardiovascular fitness. In SCI, the ability to walk is closely related to which muscle groups are spared. If quadriceps (L3 ASIA level) function is intact, then ambulation with bilateral ankle foot orthosis is possible. If the iliopsoas (L2 ASIA level) is spared, but quadriceps function is absent, a knee ankle foot orthosis (KAFO) can be fitted, and indoor ambulation is possible. However, as a practical matter, the energy cost of gait with bilateral KAFO is high, and most people will find a wheelchair more practical for community mobility. Individuals with neurological levels above L2 may walk with hip knee ankle foot orthosis (HKAFO) in the physical therapy gym. This is a form of therapeutic gait, but not a practical form of community mobility.

Paraplegia secondary to anatomical injuries at the lower lumbar vertebra (i.e., L3 burst fracture leading to cauda equina lesion) results in lower motor neuron pathology. These patients are not at risk for spasticity or detrusor sphincter dyssynergia. They will have flaccid weakness and a lower motor neuron bladder dysfunction.

Suggested Readings

Water RL, Adkins R, Yakura Y, Sie Ien. Functional and neurological recovery following acute SCI. Journal of Spinal Cord Medicine 1998; 21:195-199.

Chapter 6

Initial Rehabilitation Medicine Consultation

Shanker Nesathurai, MD, FRCP(C)
Andrew Gwardjan, MD, FRCP(C)

The purpose of this chapter is to discuss the elements of a physiatric consultation for an SCI patient. Physiatrists will usually be consulted in the acute hospital for one of three reasons. First, a new traumatically injured patient may be admitted. Second, a patient may have acute spinal cord impairment secondary to a non-traumatic cause, such as a primary tumor, metastasis, hemorrhage or infection. Third, the patient may have a remote injury, and is being readmitted for medical problems that may or may not be associated with the individual's SCI. An example of this would be a paraplegic admitted with unstable angina.

With a new injury, the patient may be admitted to the intensive care unit. At this point, the acute medical issues are most important (i.e., definitive surgical management, fluid resuscitation, etc.). However, early physiatric consultation will assist in SCI management and provide an opportunity to educate other members of the health-care team about rehabilitation care. This section will focus on the issues that a rehabilitation physician must review in the initial assessment. Many of these topics are discussed in more detail in other chapters.

Elements of a Consultation

There are certain key elements in a consultation. The consultation record should document the name and service of the consultant, as well as the name and service of the individual who requested the consultation. The chart should be thoroughly reviewed, and the pertinent history should be summarized. For a rehabilitation medicine consultation, it is important to document the patient's premorbid vocational and educational status. It is also important to determine the patient's family and home situation. For example, a patient who is a banker and lives with a caring spouse in a single-floor home has fewer discharge challenges than an unemployed, homeless patient with no family supports. A comprehensive physical examination is essential. If possible, the elements of the ASIA exam should be completed. In addition, a mental status examination as well as reflexes should be documented. The consultant's recommendations should be legible and easy to understand.

Bladder Management

Micturation requires an intact central and peripheral nervous system. Cortical and subcortical areas of the brain modulate the function of the sacral and pontine micturation centers. The bladder is innervated by sympathetic (T10 to L2, hypogastric nerve), parasympathetic (S2 to S4, pelvic nerve), and somatic (S2 to S4, pudendal nerve) fibers. If the injury affects the peripheral innervation of the bladder or completely destroys the conus medullaris, lower motor neuron bladder dysfunction may be present. If the lesion is above the sacral micturation center, the result will be an upper motor neuron bladder.

With lower motor neuron bladder dysfunction, sphincter and/or bladder tone may be absent or diminished. Patients may experience urinary incontinence or the inability to void. In the acute phase of injury, the clinical abnormalities of upper and lower motor neuron bladder dysfunction will be similar. In injuries above the sacral micturation center, the classical findings of an upper motor neuron bladder may become apparent when spinal shock resolves. Upper motor neuron bladder pathology is characterized by low urinary volumes, high bladder pressures, and uninhibited detrusor contractions. Detrusor sphincter dyssynergia (DSD) is common in lesions between the sacral and pontine micturation centers. DSD is characterized by co-contraction of the bladder and urinary sphincter. Untreated, upper motor neuron bladder dysfunction can lead to incontinence, vesicoureteral reflux, and hydronephrosis.

Most acutely injured patients will have a Foley catheter. When the patient is stable, and total urinary output is less than 3,000 cc, an intermittent catheterization program (ICP) should be started. Initially, the ICP should be on a q4 hour basis, with target volumes between 400 cc to 500 cc. If volumes are consistently small, the frequency of catheterization can be increased to q6h. The bladder management program can be individualized during the rehabilitation phase of care. Some SCI patients may be able to manage bladder dysfunction by other methods, including the Valsalva maneuver, manual suprapubic pressure (Crede maneuver), suprapubic tapping, or a condom catheter. Please refer to chapter 7 for a more detailed discussion.

Bowel Management

Most patients with upper motor neuron pathology (lesions above the conus medularis) will likely suffer from constipation. In lower motor neuron pathology, fecal incontinence is possible during acute hospitalization, although most of these patients will suffer from constipation in the post-acute phase. Narcotics and tricyclic agents may exacerbate constipation. A comprehensive bowel regimen should be instituted. In an acute injury, stool softeners, such as Colace and Senekot, can be started. The patient should be placed on the commode after breakfast to utilize the gastrocolic reflex. If obstipation is suspected, a KUB film should be obtained and a gentle enema can be considered.

Abdominal distention, pancreatitis, and gastric ulcers are possible in the acute phase of injury. The patient should be encouraged to eat when the paralytic ileus resolves. Please refer to chapter 8 for a more detailed discussion.

Pressure Ulcers

Pressure ulcers are an avoidable complication in SCI patients. The amount of time a vulnerable area is subjected to pressure should be minimized. Excessive shear forces and moisture should also be avoided. The development of an ulcer can profoundly impact the nature and length of a patient's rehabilitation care. The best way to prevent pressure ulcers is to turn and position the patient every two hours. Clinicians should monitor the skin closely. Extreme care must be used in assisted bed mobility and transfers. Maceration of the skin by urine, feces and excessive perspiration can contribute to ulcers. If there are areas of threatened skin breakdown, an alternative bed surface should be considered. Please refer to chapter 9 for a more detailed discussion.

Contractures

Immobility leads to contractures, and can be prevented. Muscles that cross two joints, such as the gastrocnemius, hamstrings, iliopsoas and biceps brachii, are at particular risk. Contractures can be prevented by passive range of movement of the joints and proper positioning (e.g., prone lying to minimize iliopsoas contractures). The physical therapy service can assist in contracture prevention. An ankle foot orthosis can prevent the progression of gastrocnemius contractures. However, an orthosis is not a substitute for a passive range of movement program. In a minority of cases, contractures should be encouraged. For example, in a patient with C6 tetraplegia, the MCP, PIP and DIP joints should be allowed to contract in approximately 20 degrees of flexion. These contractures will assist in providing a functional grasp. A volar wrist hand orthosis can help facilitate this beneficial contracture. If the spine has not been stabilized, the passive range of movement program must be approved by the surgeons to minimize any further potential spinal cord compromise. Please refer to chapter 10 for a more detailed discussion.

Autonomic Dysfunction

Patients with SCI commonly suffer from dysautonomia. In the acute phase (during spinal shock), patients may experience orthostatic hypotension, tachycardia or bradycardia. Orthostatic hypotension can be minimized by slowly elevating a patient's head and cautiously allowing the patient's legs to hang over the edge of the bed. Thigh high compression stockings and an abdominal binder can be helpful. Fludrocortisone acetate (Florinef) and ephedrine can also be used in refractory cases. Some patients will suffer from bradycardia with pulmonary suctioning due to increased vagal stimulation. In these cases, pretreatment with atropine (1 mg intravenously) and/or preoxygenation can be useful.

Disorders of temperature regulation are common in tetraplegic patients. "Quad fevers" are when SCI patients have high temperatures (i.e., above 104 degrees Fahrenheit), but have no other findings consistent with infection. These patients "look well," although they have very high body temperatures. This diagnosis should only be made when all other causes of fever have been reasonably excluded. Patients may also experience poikilothermia in which body temperature is affected by ambient temperature. Adjusting the thermostat can resolve this problem.

Autonomic dysreflexia (AD) is a syndrome characterized by headache, flushing, piloerection, hypertension and tachycardia. It is not commonly encountered in the first few weeks of SCI, but rather when a patient emerges from spinal shock. Patients with lesions above T6 are at greatest risk, although there are reports of AD with lesions below this level. **This condition is an emergency and requires immediate intervention.** If untreated, autonomic dysreflexia can lead to stroke, seizures and even death. Any noxious stimulus below the level of injury can precipitate AD. Common causes of AD include bladder distention or fecal impaction. Less common causes include pressure ulcers, ingrown toe nails, nephrolithiasis, tight clothing or heterotopic ossification. Acute abdominal pathology, such as cholecystitis or perforated viscus, can also cause autonomic dysreflexia. To manage this condition, the head should be elevated. If possible, the patient's legs should be allowed to hang from the bed in order to decrease venous return. The precipitating cause must be identified and treated. If the etiology cannot be ascertained promptly, the hypertension must be treated. A variety of agents are available, including topical nitrates, calcium channel blockers, beta blockers and centrally acting alpha agonists. Please refer to chapter 11 for a more detailed discussion.

Upper Motor Neuron Syndrome and Spasticity

Spasticity is a disorder of muscle tone characterized by a velocity dependent resistance to passive joint movement. Other manifestations of spasticity include increased muscle stretch reflexes, clonus and the "clasp-knife" phenomenon. Flexor and cutaneomotor spasms are common in upper motor neuron diseases. Although these abnormalities are not considered manifestations of spasticity, they may cause significant functional limitation. Spasms can be treated with many of the same management strategies as spasticity. Spasticity becomes more apparent as a patient emerges from spinal shock. Spasticity may be treated when it contributes to pain, impairs hygiene, interferes with nursing care, contributes to contractures, or leads to pressure ulcers. However, some patients find spasticity helpful with mobility and transfers. As such, the risks and benefits of intervention should be balanced.

Chronic SCI patients who are admitted to the hospital should remain on their spasticity medications. This is particularly important in patients who are on baclofen, as rapid withdrawal can lead to seizures, weakness and mental status changes.

Spasticity can be managed with medications such as baclofen (Lioresal), tizanidine (Zanaflex), diazepam (Valium), dantrolene sodium (Dantrium), and clonidine (Catapres). Other interventions include motor branch blocks, nerve blocks and botulinum toxin injections. In refractory cases, an intrathecal baclofen pump can be considered. Please refer to chapter 12 for a more detailed discussion.

DVT Prophylaxis

SCI patients are at very high risk for developing deep venous thrombosis (DVT). As DVT can lead to pulmonary emboli and potentially death, prophylaxis is essential. The therapeutic options include intermittent pneumatic compression devices (e.g., Venodyne boots), thigh high graded compression stockings (e.g., TED stockings), coumadin, minidose subcutaneous unfractionated heparin (5,000 units bid), adjusted dose subcutaneous unfractionated heparin, or low molecular weight heparin. A Greenfield filter also may be indicated in selected cases. If there are no contraindications to low molecular weight heparin (i.e., active bleeding, profound thrombocytopenia, etc.), then enoxaparin (Lovenox) may be the best intervention to prevent DVT. However, some surgeons and critical care physicians are concerned about potential bleeding in the spinal cord and are hesitant to start anticoagulants in the acute phase of injury. When there are strong reservations about low molecular weight heparin, utilization of intermittent compression devices and compression stockings in addition to serial doppler surveillance may be a reasonable compromise. However, serial doppler studies are expensive and fail to detect a significant number of calf thrombosis. In high risk patients (i.e., complete high quadriplegia with femur fracture) where enoxoparin cannot be prescribed, a Greenfield filter may be considered. Later, in the rehabilitation phase of management, low molecular weight heparin can be instituted.

Pulmonary Issues

Normal ventilation requires the diaphragm (C3 to C5), intercostal (T1 to T12), upper abdominal muscles (T8 to T10), and lower abdominal muscles (T10 to T12). Tetraplegics may have paralysis of the intercostal and abdominal muscles. In tetraplegia, the accessory muscles of ventilation, such as scalene anticus, scalene medius, levator scapula and trapezius, are usually spared. These muscles are essential for ventilation. Intercostal and abdominal muscle paralysis results in an impaired cough and subsequent difficulty clearing secretions. Pneumonia is commonly encountered. Aggressive chest physical therapy techniques, such as assisted cough ("quad cough"), chest wall percussion, breath stacking, and postural draining positioning, may decrease secretions and mucus plugging.

High tetraplegics (i.e., those with lesions above C4) many times are unable to be weaned off the ventilator. These patients will require tracheostomy and long-term ventilation. High tetraplegics who have some intact lower motor neuron supply to the diaphragm may benefit from "pacing" the phrenic nerve. With this intervention, some high tetraplegics may be liberated from a ventilator for some part of the day.

Psychological Adaptation

Patients with catastrophic SCI may experience a range of emotions, including denial, anger, guilt, disbelief and frustration. There is no "normal" pattern of coping. Families also may require emotional and psychological support. The rehabilitation psychology, social work and pastoral care services may provide comfort and support. These services should be consulted early in SCI. Please refer to chapter 14 for a more detailed discussion.

Pain

Patients with acute lesions can experience significant pain. Pain should be treated with judicious use of narcotic and non-narcotic analgesics. Many patients complain of neuropathic pain which may be manifested by poorly localized dysesthesias. This can be treated with low dose tricyclic agents, such as amitriptyline (Elavil), nortriptyline (Pamelor), or imipramine (Tofranil). These agents have anticholinergic side effects such as dry mouth, light headedness, blurred vision, and orthostatic hypotension. Anti-seizure medications may also palliate neuropathic pain, including carbamazepine (Tegretol), gabapentin (Neurontin), and phenytoin (Dilantin). Non-pharmacological interventions to control pain include transcutaneous electrical nerve stimulation (TENS) and acupuncture. Psychological pain managment techniques can be considered, including hypnosis and relaxation therapy.

In chronic spinal cord patients who are admitted for concurrent surgical procedures, adequate pain relief is essential. Autonomic dysreflexia and increased spasticity can be precipitated by untreated pain.

Comorbid Conditions.

Many persons with SCI have other injuries such as fractures, abdominal wounds, traumatic brain injuries, seizure disorders, pneumothorax, cardiac contusions, and peripheral nerve injuries. Some patients also have substance abuse disorders. These co-existing impairments must be documented in the consultation record. Comorbid conditions could affect the rehabilitation care a patient requires. For example, a patient with an L5 paraplegia should be able to walk with braces. However, if the injured individual also has an acetabular fracture, he may not be permitted to bear weight for many weeks. As such, wheelchair-level goals would be appropriate for this patient.

SCI can be associated with concomitant head injuries. Sometimes, traumatic brain injuries (TBI) are unrecognized due to relative subtle deficits or normal neuroimaging. A negative CT scan or MRI of the brain, however, does not exclude a traumatic brain injury. A mental status exam should be completed whenever possible. If there is a high index of suspicion, a neuropsychological consultation should be obtained.

Patients with TBI and SCI present a unique challenge to the rehabilitation team. The team will have to manage the sequelae of TBI (agitation, memory impairments, attention deficits) in addition to SCI issues. More resources will be required to achieve equal functional gains with a dually diagnosed patient.

Disposition and Discharge Planning

Discharge planning should begin as soon as the patient is admitted to the hospital. Physiatrists should advocate for appropriate comprehensive spinal cord injury care. Institutions with SCI programs certified by the Commission on the Accreditation of Rehabilitation Facilities (CARF) or designated as National Model Spinal Cord Injury System Centers will probably provide excellent care. Insurance carriers may compel patients to receive rehabilitation services from "preferred" providers. Some patients will request rehabilitation services at sites close to their homes or for other personal reasons.

Long-Term Issues

During the initial consultation, it is important to consider long-term issues. This is particularly true for a patient with a remote SCI. Every patient must be encouraged to locate a primary care physician who is knowledgeable about spinal cord medicine. Healthcare services should be available in an architecturally accessible facility. Physiatrists should encourage patients to participate in routine health maintenance (e.g., screening for cancer and cardiovascular disease, updating immunizations, etc.). Long-term issues are discussed in more detail in chapter 16.

Checklist for Acute Spinal Cord Injury Rehabilitation Medicine Consultation

- Detailed Clinical Summary of Injury
- Document Comorbid Conditions
- Comprehensive Physical Examination
- Document ASIA Assessment

Comment on the Following Issues

- Bladder
- Bowel
- Pressure Ulcers
- Contracture Prevention
- Dysautonomia
- Spasticity
- Psychological Adaptation
- DVT Prophylaxis
- Pulmonary
- Pain
- Comorbid Conditions
- Disposition and Discharge Planning
- Long-Term Issues

Suggested Readings

Yarkony GM, Chen D. Rehabilitation of patients with spinal cord injuries. In: Braddom RL. Physical Medicine & Rehabilitation. Philadelphia: W.B. Saunders Company; 1996; 1149-1179.

Freed MM. Traumatic and congenital lesions of the spinal cord. In: Kottke FJ, Lehmann JF. Krusen's handbook of rehabilitation medicine. 4th ed. Philadelphia: W.B. Saunders Company; 1990; 717-748.

Chapter 7

Bladder Management

Shanker Nesathurai, MD, FRCP(C)

Introduction

The mortality and morbidity associated with urological disease is significant in the SCI population. After World War II, renal failure was the leading cause of death in persons with SCI. With advances in urological management, renal pathology is now the fourth leading cause of death.

The two major functions of the bladder are storage and emptying of urine. This complex activity requires the coordinated function of the peripheral nervous system, sacral micturition center, pontine micturition center, and the cerebral cortex. In infants, voiding is not meaningfully influenced by the cortex, and voiding is initiated reflexively in response to bladder fullness. In adults, the pontine micturition center is modulated by higher centers, which facilitate voiding at socially appropriate times.

Innervation of the Lower Urinary Tract

The lower urinary tract is innervated by the somatic, parasympathetic and sympathetic nervous systems. The somatic nuclei are located in the anterior horn of the gray matter of the S2 to S4 spinal cord. These fibers project through the pudendal nerve to innervate the external urethral sphincter (striated muscle). Preganglionic parasympathetic neurons originate in the intermediolateral horn of the gray matter of the S2 to S4 segments. These fibers travel through the pelvic nerves to the prostatic plexus. Postganglionic parasympathetic fibers originating in the prostatic plexus then supply the detrusor of the bladder. Increasing parasympathetic tone will facilitate detrusor contraction and voiding. The sympathetic (alpha and beta adrenergic) fibers originate in the T10 to L2 spinal segments and project through the sympathetic chain and inferior mesenteric ganglion. These neurons travel to the bladder via the hypogastric nerve. The alpha adrenergic sympathetic neurons supply the bladder neck (internal sphincter). The stimulation of alpha adrenergic nerves will cause contraction of the bladder neck; this is the primary mechanism that promotes urinary continence and prevents retrograde ejaculation. Beta adrenergic stimulation will inhibit detrusor contraction and assist in urinary storage.

Spinal Tracts Affecting Bladder Function

Sensory impulses from the proprioceptive nerve endings in the mucosal wall of the bladder, abdominal wall, urethra and periurethral areas travel through the lateral somatic and posterior columns in the spinal cord. These impulses are relayed to different areas of the brain. Motor control of bladder and sphincter function is modulated by the descending bulbospinal, reticulospinal and cerulospinal tracts.

Coordination of Micturition

The pontine micturition center coordinates contraction and relaxation of the detrusor and sphincter. During urination, the detrusor muscle contracts after the sphincter relaxes. During storage, the opposite must occur; the detrusor muscle must relax while the sphincter contracts (guarding reflex). This coordination of the contraction and relaxation is called detrusor sphincter synergia.

The medial frontal lobe, corpus callosum, limbic system, hypothalamus, basal ganglia and cerebellum are all involved in the control of bladder function. They exert either facilitatory or inhibitory influences upon the bladder by projecting impulses through the pontine micturition center or directly to the sacral segments.

Medical and Social Issues Related to SCI Bladder Management

Clinicians must be sensitive to both the medical and social issues related to SCI bladder dysfunction. From a medical perspective, the primary goal is to preserve renal function. Repeated upper urinary tract infections and vesicoureteral reflux will contribute to renal scarring and progressive renal failure. In addition, urinary incontinence can cause skin maceration, which can contribute to skin breakdown.

Bladder dysfunction has significant social consequences. Frequently, the injured person will have urinary incontinence. Some patients may have to rely on others for catheterization or for the cleaning of soiled bed linens and clothing. This may result in personal embarrassment. These feelings can be compounded if family members must perform these tasks.

Lower Motor Neuron Bladder Dysfunction

Bladder dysfunction is closely related to the level of the injury. If the lesion involves exclusively the peripheral innervation of the bladder or completely destroys the sacral micturation center, the result is a lower motor neuron bladder. This type of bladder pathology may be associated with a hypotonic detrusor and/or sphincter. Consequently, clinical findings include urinary retention with associated overflow incontinence. Alternatively, incontinence may be secondary to diminished sphincter tone.

Upper Motor Neuron Bladder Dysfunction and Detrusor Sphincter Dyssynergia

If the injury is above the sacral micturation center, the result is an upper motor neuron bladder; this type of dysfunction is characterized by low urinary volumes, high bladder pressures, bladder trabeculation, and diminished bladder compliance. In some cases, uninhibited detrusor contractions ("bladder spasms") may trigger autonomic dysreflexia. Most patients with upper motor neuron bladders will have some incontinence. Many patients (perhaps more than 85 percent) with SCI develop detrusor sphincter dyssynergia (DSD). This condition is common in neurological injuries between the sacral and pontine micturation center. DSD is characterized by co-contraction of the bladder and sphincter.

Vesicoureteral Reflux

The distal portion of the ureter enters into the bladder at an oblique angle, and the ureteral meatus opens at the posterolateral portion of the trigone. Increased intravesical pressure will usually compress the submucosal portion of the ureter against the detrusor muscle, thus obliterating the ureter. Because of this valve mechanism, vesicoureteral reflux (VUR) is absent in adults. The effectiveness of this valve mechanism depends on the ratio of ureteral diameter to the length of the submucosal ureter.

The bladder is able to eliminate urine only when the intravesical pressure exceeds the urethral pressure. Therefore, voiding may be incomplete with DSD. The urine remaining in the bladder is the post void residual (PVR) volume. High PVR (perhaps greater than 100 cc) with high intravesical pressures may be associated with vesicoureteral reflux. In this case, with bladder contraction, some of the urine travels through the incompetent ureter-bladder valve mechanism and into the kidneys.

There is no consensus on absolute intravesical pressure that will lead to VUR. Intravesical pressures of 40 cm to 60 cm of water may be associated with VUR. The diagnosis of VUR may be confirmed by a voiding cystogram.

Figure 7.1 **Typical Urodynamic Study**

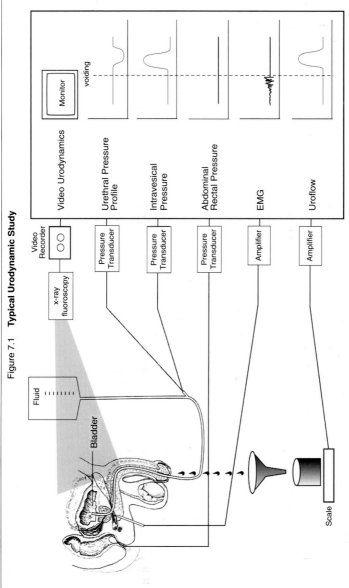

Instrumentation for urodynamic studies is not standardized. The illustration above uses radio-opaque fluid. Some physicians, however, prefer to use carbon dioxide. Normal bladder function can be divided into storage and voiding phases. The first sensation of bladder filling is between 100 cc and 200 cc. The patient experiences bladder fullness between 300 cc and 400 cc and the sense of urgency between 400 cc and 500 cc. Intravesical pressure does not increase significantly during the storage phase due to the vascoelasticity of the vesical wall. During the voiding phase, sphincter activity stops and the bladder contracts. During normal voiding, the EMG signal will be silent, intravesical pressure will increase, and urethral pressure will decrease. Fluoroscopy will qualitatively assess bladder contraction and document any potential vesicoureteral reflux.

47

Urodynamic Studies

Urodynamic studies (Figure 7.1) are important in assessing the nature of voiding function. However, this study must be utilized in conjunction with good clinical judgment and may have some limitations. Urodynamic findings may change from the acute phase of injury to the chronic phase. This is especially true in upper motor neuron and mixed lesions. Arguably, the test is unphysiological; many times, the bladder is filled with gas through the urethra at an unphysiological rate. With physiological urological function, the bladder is filled slowly through the ureters with fluid. Psychological stress can also affect urodynamic findings, especially the initiation of voiding. In addition, a urodynamic study is a sample of a single storage-voiding cycle and may not be representative of the bladder being tested. Finally, the results can be affected by the instrumentation, type of catheter used, and the position of the patient during testing.

Management of Lower Motor Neuron Bladder Dysfunction

This type of bladder pathology will result in two possible clinical scenarios. In the first scenario, sphincter tone is diminished; however, detrusor tone is normal or compromised. This individual will have continuous incontinence. For a male patient, a condom catheter will be satisfactory. In a female patient, an indwelling catheter will be required. Theoretically, sphincter tone can be increased with alpha adrenergic medications (i.e., ephedrine). However, as a practical matter, this is unlikely to result in socially acceptable continence. In selected cases, an artificial sphincter may permit continence. The second scenario is where the sphincter is competent to maintain acceptable continence, but bladder tone is diminished and the individual cannot micturate. In this scenario, an intermittent catheterization program (ICP) can be recommended. Another alternative is bladder evacuation with the Valsava maneuver or suprapubic pressure (Crede maneuver). An indwelling catheter is a less satisfactory treatment for this type of bladder dysfunction. Cholinergic agonists such as bethanechol chloride (Urecholine) are ineffective in increasing detrusor tone in SCI.

Management of Upper Motor Neuron Bladder Dysfunction

During spinal shock, patients with upper motor neuron and lower motor neuron bladder dysfunction will have similar clinical abnormalities. Consequently, the management strategies will be similar.

As spinal shock resolves, the manifestations of an upper motor neuron bladder will become evident. Most patients with upper motor neuron bladder dysfunction will have some incontinence. At this stage, a urodynamic study will assist in clarifying the nature of voiding function.

Medications with anticholinergic properties—oxybutynin, imipramine, propantheline bromide—will decrease detrusor tone and allow for greater bladder capacity (Table 1). This intervention may also reduce VUR and uninhibited bladder contractions. SCI patients with upper motor neuron bladder dysfunction who are able to engage in an ICP may benefit from this intervention. As well, a few persons with incomplete or mixed lesions may utilize suprapubic tapping in conjunction with anticholinergic medications.

On rare occasions, bladder augmentation can increase bladder capacity. This is a surgical procedure that increases vesical volume by interposing a piece of small bowel with bladder tissue. The patient can then engage in an ICP. A competent sphincter is required for this bladder management strategy.

Patients who have upper motor neuron bladders and are unable to use an ICP will require an indwelling catheter (preferably a suprapubic tube). In male patients, an alternative management strategy could be a complete sphincterotomy, which would lead to continuous incontinence. A condom catheter could then be employed.

Micturation requires detrusor pressures to exceed bladder outlet pressures. Some individuals with SCI may not be able to void as a result of increased internal sphincter tone. Medications and procedures may successfully decrease outlet obstruction and thereby allow voiding with suprapubic tapping, Valsava maneuver or manual suprapubic pressure (Crede maneuver). Alpha adrenergic antagonists, such as terazosin, prazosin doxazosin or tamsulosin, may decrease internal sphincter tone (Table 2). However, these medications may cause significant hypotension, and the doses should be carefully titrated. In men, a sphincterotomy which moderately decreases outlet obstruction may improve bladder emptying. However, many patients are rendered incontinent and will require a condom catheter. Other side effects include bleeding and loss of erectile function. Recurrence of urinary obstruction may occur due to fibrosis and subsequent procedures may be required. In male patients, external sphincter tone can be decreased with transuretheral or transperineal botulinum toxin. This procedure is not recommended in women as it may result in incontinence. The effects of botulinum toxin range from three to six months. To decrease external sphincter tone (striated muscle), baclofen, diazepam and dantrolene may be considered; however, these medications are usually unsuccessful.

Table 1
Medications With Anticholinergic Properties That Decrease Bladder Tone

Medication	Brand Name	Initial Dose	Maximum Dose	Precautions
oxybutynin chloride	Ditropan	5 mg bid	5 mg qid	dry mouth blurred vision rash nausea vomiting sedation tachycardia urinary retention constipation
imipramine hcl	Tofranil	25 mg tid	50 mg tid	dry mouth blurred vision sedation tachycardia nausea vomiting orthostatic hypotension photosensitivity
propantheline bromide	Pro-Banthine	7.5 mg tid	30 mg tid and qhs	dry mouth blurred vision palpitations headache sedation

Table 2
Medications That Reduce Urethral Outflow Resistance

Medication	Brand Name	Initial Dose	Maximum Dose	Mechanism	Precautions
terazosin	Hytrin	1mg qhs	5 mg bid	alpha-1 antagonist	hypotension sedation headaches syncope
doxazosin	Cardura	1mg qd	16 mg qd	alpha-1 antagonist	hypotension sedation headache snycope
tamsulosin	Flomax	0.4 mg qd	0.8 mg qd	alpha-1A antagonist	no significant hypotension in non-SCI patients retrograde ejaculation nausea diarrhea headache
prazosin	Minipress	1 mg bid	5 mg tid	alpha-1 antagonist	hypotension sedation headache

Guidelines for an Intermittent Catheterization Program

Many times, an intermittent catheterization program (ICP) is the preferred method of treating bladder dysfunction. An ICP may be started when the patient is medically stable and daily urine output is less than 3,000 cc. ICP should be initiated at four- or six-hour intervals. Acceptable catheterization volumes should not exceed 400 cc to 500 cc. Larger amounts may result in bladder distention and excessive intravesical pressure. The primary method of regulating urinary output is fluid intake. Persons with SCI should be encouraged to adjust fluid consumption accordingly in order to minimize excessive catheterization volumes. A detailed diary of fluid intake and catheter volumes should be maintained.

A four-times-a-day ICP is more practical than a strict every-six-hour program; a strict every-six-hour program would require waking the person with SCI during the night. In addition, those individuals who cannot perform self-catheterization may have difficulty finding a caregiver to perform intermittent catheterization during the night. Nighttime catheterization, if required, should be coordinated with the turning schedule for skin protection. Clinicians should discuss these issues with patients and prospective caregivers.

Persons with SCI who perform self-catheterization may utilize a clean technique. Sterile catheterization is not required. The terminal end of the urethra is colonized by normal flora in all individuals. Even with strict sterile catheterization, these microorganisms will be introduced into the bladder.

50

Many tetraplegics do not have adequate upper extremity function to independently perform intermittent self-catheterization or other tasks associated with bladder management (i.e., undressing, transfers, disposing of urine, etc.). In some cases, a less than optimal bladder management program is provided because of the lack of human or financial resources. For example, a C5 tetraplegic may benefit from an ICP; however, if a competent caregiver is unavailable to perform the procedure, then other bladder management strategies must be considered.

Indwelling Catheter

A less ideal alternative to an ICP is an indwelling catheter such as a Foley or suprapubic tube. An indwelling catheter is indicated for an individual who is unable or unwilling to engage in an ICP. Some individuals who have vesicoureteral reflux or significant incontinence refractory to other treatment strategies may also benefit from an indwelling catheter. Foley catheters are associated with bladder stones, prostatitis and epididymitis, as well as urethral strictures. An indwelling catheter should be changed every four weeks. A suprapubic tube is preferred, as the incidence of epididymitis and prostatitis are decreased. Sexual intercourse is more easily facilitated with a suprapubic tube when compared with a Foley catheter. As individuals with indwelling catheters (both Foley and suprapubic) have an increased risk of transitional cell and squamous cell carcinoma of the bladder, a cystoscopy every two years is recommended.

Clamping of the Foley

Clamping of the Foley catheter has been advocated as a method of "bladder retraining." This intervention is not recommended, as it may lead to overdistention of the bladder, contribute to urinary tract infections, and may precipitate autonomic dysreflexia.

Pathophysiology of Urinary Tract Infection

Urinary tract infections (UTI) are generally caused by the endogenous flora of the host overcoming other competing normal flora and host defense mechanisms. The presence of the urinary tract infection is affected by the virulence of the invading microorganism, the condition of the urine as the culture medium, and the host defense mechanisms. In healthy individuals, there is a critical balance between the microorganism virulence factors and host defense mechanisms. These virulence factors become less important when the host defense mechanisms are compromised by catheterization or immunosuppression.

Colonization is the growth of microorganisms in the urine without tissue invasion. In contrast, a urinary tract infection is the microbial colonization of urine with associated tissue invasion of the uroepithelium. Persons with SCI are at risk for UTI for a number of reasons. Many individuals are colonized with nosocomial organisms. In addition, elevated post void residual urinary volumes favor bacterial growth. ICP programs introduce bacterial flora from the urethra on a regular basis. A few patients are immunocompromised.

Many common urinary pathogens (i.e., E. Coli or Proteus) possess surface projections known as fimbriae. These projections adhere to the uroepithelium and increase the virulence of the organism. Some bacteria also contain extracellular proteins that resist phagocytosis.

In general, an acidic concentrated urine inhibits microbial growth. Urinary tract infections are prevented by the "wash out" effect of large volumes of urine. The large flow of fluid impedes the adherence of microorganisms and dilutes the concentration of microorganisms. However, large fluid volumes may decrease urine osmolarity, which favors bacterial growth. In addition, excessive fluids may complicate an intermittent catheterization program. Other defenses against UTI include the mucin coat and Taumm-Horfall proteins produced in the bladder. Furthermore, IgM, IgA and IgG antibodies secreted by the kidneys provide some added protection.

Management of Symptomatic UTI

UTI can present with many of the following symptoms: fever, increased spasticity, foul smelling urine, frequency, dysuria or urinary incontinence. When UTI is diagnosed on the basis of the clinical presentation and urinalysis abnormalities, antibiotic treatment can be instituted after sending a sample to the laboratory for a culture and sensitivity. A five- to seven-day course of oral treatment is sufficient for uncomplicated lower tract infections. Symptomatic reinfections may require a longer course of treatment. If the UTI is complicated by sepsis, intravenous antibiotics are required. A Foley catheter may be temporarily instituted if fluid intake is excessive and results in unacceptable intermittent catheterization volumes.

Asymptomatic UTI

Maintaining sterile urine at all times in the SCI population is not feasible. Treating asymptomatic UTI may result in colonization with even more virulent drug resistant organisms. In general, asymptomatic UTI in individuals with indwelling catheters should not be treated. If an ICP is utilized, an asymptomatic UTI with less than 50 white blood cells per high-power field should not be treated unless there is evidence of vesicoureteral reflux, hydronephrosis, or growth of urea splitting organisms.

Prophylactic Treatment

The role of prophylactic antibiotics has not been established. Methenamine salts, vitamin C supplementation, and cranberry juice can acidify the urine. However, these interventions have not been demonstrated to be effective prophylactic agents in controlled studies.

Suggested Reading

Krane RJ, Siroky MB. Clinical neuro-urology. Boston: Little Brown and Company; 1991.

Chapter 8

Bowel Management

Susan Biener Bergman, MD

Introduction

Bowel dysfunction in SCI is a major source of morbidity. SCI patients require a bowel program that allows for socially acceptable continence and prevents fecal impaction. This chapter reviews the pathophysiologic basis of normal and SCI-related bowel dysfunction. Treatment strategies will also be discussed.

Anatomy and Physiology of the Gastrointestinal Tract

The main function of the gastrointestinal (Figure 8.1) tract is to provide the body with water, nutrients and electrolytes. Food is ingested and mechanically and chemically processed in the mouth. It is digested in the stomach and further processed in the small intestine. Digestive end products are then absorbed in the small intestine and the proximal half of the colon. The colon functions as both a storage area and a processing center for waste products as food moves through the GI tract. It is responsible for the absorption of water, electrolytes and short chain fatty acids from the stool. It also supports the growth of beneficial bacteria, secretes mucus to lubricate the stool, and pushes stool out of the body through the rectum and anus.

The colon is essentially a closed tube that is bound proximally by the ileocecal valve and distally by the anal sphincter. It is composed of smooth muscle oriented in an inner circular and an outer longitudinal layer. In between these layers lies Auerbach's plexus and Meissner's plexus, which provide part of the colon's intrinsic innervation. At the end of the colon, at the rectum, the smooth muscle layers thicken to form the internal anal sphincter (IAS). The external anal sphincter (EAS) consists of a circular band of striated muscle that is part of the pelvic floor. The colon and pelvic floor muscles receive parasympathetic, sympathetic and somatic nerve supply.

The parasympathetic supply to the gut consists of both cranial (vagus nerve) and sacral (pelvic nerve) divisions. In general, increased parasympathetic tone stimulates the gut wall. Sympathetic innervation of the gut projects through the hypogastric nerve via the superior mesenteric, inferior mesenteric, and celiac ganglia. Sympathetic stimulation relaxes the gut wall, ileocecal valve and the IAS. Somatic nerve supply comes from the pudendal nerve (S2 to S4), which supplies the EAS and the pelvic floor musculature.

Intrinsic innervation of the gut is provided by the myenteric plexus (Auerbach's plexus), which lies between the muscle layers and serves primarily a motor function, and the submucosal plexus (Meissner's plexus), which serves primarily a sensory function. Stimulating the myenteric plexus increases the activity of the gut, including increased force and velocity of contractions. The submucosal plexus plays an important role in coordinating gut wall movements, as well as the secretion of digestive juices.

Two types of movements occur in the digestive tract and are equally important: mixing movements, which agitate intestinal contents and facilitate extraction of nutrients, and peristaltic movements to propel the food bolus toward the rectum and out of the body when the extraction process is complete. Coordination of these movements takes place by three mechanisms: chemical control via neurotransmitters and hormones (i.e., substance P, gastrin and cholecystikinin), neurogenic control via the enteric reflexes (i.e., gastrocolic and rectocolic reflexes), and myenteric control. Since individual smooth muscle fibers in the gut lie very close to one another and some of the membranes are actually fused, the fibers can function as a syncytium through which electrical signals are easily propagated from one fiber to the next. Colonic movements can either involve large sections of the gut (peristalsis), or they can be relatively localized (mixing movements).

Defecation in the Neurologically Intact Individual

The defecation process normally starts when stool is pushed into the rectum by peristalsis. The volume of stool stretches the puborectalis muscle as well as the rectal wall, stimulating the urge to defecate. Voluntary relaxation of the external anal sphincter and the puborectalis muscle straighten the anorectum, allowing for the passage of stool. Stool is pushed out with a combination of continued peristalsis and increased intra-abdominal pressure via the Valsalva maneuver.

Defecation in the Spinal Cord Injured Individual

The SCI individual typically loses both the sensation of rectal fullness and the ability to voluntarily relax the EAS. Depending on the level and completeness of the injury, one of two patterns of bowel dysfunction is seen. In lesions above the conus medullaris, an upper motor neuron (hyperreflexic) bowel is present. The EAS cannot be voluntarily relaxed and the pelvic floor muscles become spastic. However, nerve connections between the spinal cord and colon, as well as the myenteric plexus, remain intact and the stool can be propelled by reflex activity. In lesions below the conus medullaris, a lower motor neuron (areflexic) bowel is present. The myenteric plexus coordinates the movement of stool, but it tends to be quite slow. Most SCI patients experience constipation and, on occasion, fecal impaction. Fecal incontinence is relatively infrequent.

Management of Neurogenic Bowel Dysfunction in Spinal Cord Injury

Although the goals of a treatment plan must be individualized for each patient, the following is a general discussion of a reasonable bowel care program. Prior to instituting a bowel program, premorbid and current bowel function must be ascertained. Preexisting conditions, including laxative dependency, autonomic neuropathy (i.e., secondary to diabetes), irritable bowel syndrome, or inflammatory bowel disease, may alter gut transit time. These diseases may also diminish the effectiveness of bowel care medications.

For most patients, a complete bowel evacuation every other day is satisfactory. Less frequent bowel movements may result in fecal impaction. For most tetraplegics, a caregiver is needed to complete the bowel regimen. Furthermore, a bowel evacuation may take up to two hours to complete. As such, the bowel program must be scheduled at a time convenient to both patient and caregiver.

When initiating a bowel program, it is worthwhile to begin with an empty gut. A plain X-ray of the abdomen can be helpful. If obstipation is present, an enema should precede the beginning of the bowel program.

Medications that decrease bowel motility, such as tricyclic agents or narcotics, should be minimized. Broad spectrum antibiotics may inadvertently alter gut flora and result in diarrhea. In such cases, consumption of yogurt or lactobacillus preparations (i.e., Lactinex) restore normal gut flora.

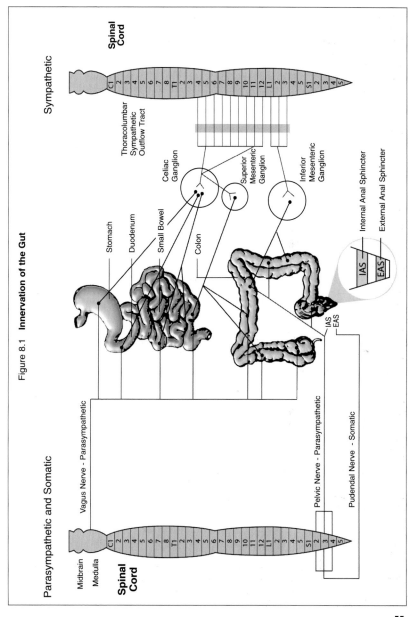

Figure 8.1 **Innervation of the Gut**

Parasympathetic and Somatic

Midbrain
Medulla
Spinal Cord

Vagus Nerve - Parasympathetic

Pelvic Nerve - Parasympathetic

Pudendal Nerve - Somatic

Sympathetic

Thoracolumbar Sympathetic Outflow Tract

Spinal Cord

Celiac Ganglion

Superior Mesenteric Ganglion

Inferior Mesenteric Ganglion

Stomach
Duodenum
Small Bowel
Colon

IAS
EAS

IAS Internal Anal Sphincter
EAS External Anal Sphincter

Diet

Proper diet is an integral part of successful overall bowel management. Soft bulky stools are more likely to decrease bowel transit time. Toward this goal, the diet should contain adequate amounts of fluids and fiber. Caffeinated beverages, prune juice and apricot nectar can also aid in bowel evacuation. Fatty foods and dairy products, in general, will decrease bowel transit time.

"Fiber" refers to a variety of poorly digestible components of plant material, primarily carbohydrates. There are different types of fiber, which have differing effects on the gastrointestinal tract. The specific effect depends on the degree of water solubility, as well as the location along the GI tract. In the stomach, dietary fiber tends to prolong gastric emptying time. In the small intestine, fiber can delay absorption of nutrients as well as promote or inhibit stool transit. In the colon, fiber tends to shorten transit time. It provides bulk to stool and eases the transit along the lower bowel, increasing the frequency of bowel movements. This effect is more pronounced with coarsely ground fiber. Good sources of fiber include whole grain breads and bran cereals. Wheat germ can be added to foods to boost fiber intake if bran cereals are not palatable to the patient. Fruits and vegetables can also provide fiber as well as fluid. An added benefit of a high fiber diet is a feeling of satiety, which may limit the intake of high fat foods.

A careful diet history must be taken to determine the baseline amount of fiber intake. A total of 15 grams of dietary fiber a day from a variety of sources is probably ideal. This target amount should be achieved gradually. Patients must be closely monitored for any symptoms of intolerance such as unacceptable flatulence, significantly increased stool volume, and painful abdominal distention.

Fluid Intake

Adequate fluid intake (2,500 cc to 3,000 cc per day is ideal) is also essential to a good bowel program. The recommended fluid intake, however, must also be consistent with the bladder management program.

Adjunctive Medications

There are five main classes of medications used to modify bowel habits: stool softeners, colonic stimulants, colonic (contact) irritants, bulk formers, and prokinetic agents (Table 1). The introduction of medications should be individualized. However, stool sof-

Table 1
Sample Oral Adjunctive Bowel Medications

Medication	Brand	Mechanism of Action	Strength	Dose
docusate sodium	Colace	stool softener	100 mg caps	i-ii bid
senna	Senokot	colonic stimulant	187 mg tabs	ii qd
bisacodyl	Dulcolax	colonic irritant	5 mg tabs	ii qd
psyllium powder	Metamucil	bulk forming agent	3.4 mg per tsp	i tsp qd-tid
metoclopramide	Reglan	prokinetic agent	10 mg tabs	i qid

teners prevent the formation of hard stools and should be the first-line medication. This should make bowel evacuation easier.

Glycerin and bisacodyl (Dulcolax) suppositories can be useful adjunctive agents in a bowel regimen. Enemas (e.g., Fleet, Soap Suds) should not be part of a regular bowel program; however, these agents are useful in providing a clear gut prior to beginning a bowel program or for treating fecal obstipation.

Gastrocolic and Rectocolic Reflex

Gastrocolic and rectocolic reflexes can be helpful in managing bowel and upper motor neuron bowel dysfunction. The gastrocolic reflex is a normal phenomenon that results in defecation after eating a meal. As such, SCI patients should be placed on the commode within one hour subsequent to a meal. The rectocolic reflex can be manipulated by digital stimulation of the rectum. Digital stimulation is accomplished by gently inserting a lubricated finger into the rectum, and slowly moving the digit in a clockwise manner. A suppository may also be helpful.

Equipment and Positioning

The best position for elimination is sitting upright with the hips and knees flexed on a commode. If possible, the feet should be slightly elevated to place the knees slightly higher than the hips. A less optimal position is the left lateral position in bed. These positions allow for gravity to assist in the flow of stool and places the abdominal muscles at maximum mechanical advantage. A shower commode or patient lift may be required. Care must be taken to prevent pressure ulcers, regardless of whether the bowel evacuation is completed in the bed or on a commode.

Basic Bowel Care Plan for New SCI Patient

- Complete history and physical examination
- Determine goals of bowel program (frequency, timing, location)
- Minimize medications that may decrease bowel motility
- Recommend diet high in fiber, fruits and vegetables
- Minimize fatty foods and dairy products, which may impair gut motility
- KUB to ensure unobstructed bowel
- Introduce stool softener
- Place patient on commode after breakfast to manipulate gastrocolic reflex
- Encourage defecation in sitting position, not in bed
- If no bowel movement, then perform rectal stimulation. If this is unsuccessful, consider suppository
- If no bowel movement after third day, give enema and consider adding second adjunctive medication

Fecal Impaction

The goal of a good bowel regimen is to prevent fecal impaction, which is characterized by absent or diminished passage of stool. Sometimes, overflow diarrhea can be present. Impaction can trigger autonomic dysreflexia, or even lead to a perforated viscus. If impacted stool is present in the rectum, manual disimpaction should be attempted. Anesthetic jelly should be used to prevent autonomic dysreflexia. If the impaction is more proximal, enemas or potent oral stimulants (e.g., magnesium citrate) may be indicated. Surgical consultation may also be indicated. In cases of repeated fecal impaction associated with multiple episodes of dysreflexia, ileostomy or colostomy may be indicated.

Hemorrhoids

Hemorrhoids are usually caused by increased rectal pressure and are often associated with prolonged efforts to remove hard stools. Suppositories, enemas or digital stimulation may exacerbate hemorrhoids. Symptoms include bleeding, pain and autonomic dysreflexia. Effective treatment strategies include maintaining soft stools and regular bowel movements. Topical steroid ointments and medicated suppositories are effective in treating symptoms. If hemorrhoids do not respond to these interventions, then surgical consultation is warranted.

Neurogenic Bowel Across the Lifespan

As in the general population, remaining active and maintaining an optimal level of fitness may also help achieve regular and predictable bowel emptying. Aside from lifestyle issues, establishing and maintaining a regular bowel regime will reduce the risk of chronic GI problems, including fecal impaction, hemorrhoids, gastroesophageal reflux disorder, and diverticulosis.

SCI patients are living longer and suffering from many of the diseases that afflict the healthy community, including duodenal ulcers and diverticulitis. Patients may also develop upper and lower gastrointestinal tract malignancies. Physicians should screen all patients over age 50, including those with SCI, for colorectal cancers with fecal occult blood tests and colonoscopy.

Suggested Readings

Banwell JG, Creasey GH, Aggarwal AM, Mortimer JT. Management of the neurogenic bowel in patients with spinal cord injury. Urologic Clinics of North America 1993 August; 20 (3):517-526.

Consortium for Spinal Cord Medicine. Neurogenic bowel management in adults with spinal cord injury. Clinical Practice Guidelines 1998; Paralyzed Veterans Association.

Frost FS. Gastrointestinal dysfunction in spinal cord injury. In Yarkony GM. Spinal cord injury: medical management and rehabilitation. Gaithersburg, MD: Aspen; 1994.

Steins SA, Bergman SB, Goetz LL. Neurogenic bowel dysfunction after spinal cord injury: clinical evaluation and rehabilitative management. (Review) Arch Physical Medicine and Rehabilitation 78 (1997): S86 - S102.

Walker-Dalton LM. Bowel care: implementing changes toward quality improvement. SCI Nursing 1995 March; 12 (1): 8-9.

Chapter 9

Pressure Ulcers

Mary Glover, MS, RNC

Overview

The SCI population is at significant risk for pressure ulcers. It is estimated that up to 80 percent of SCI individuals will experience a pressure ulcer during their lifetime, and 30 percent will experience recurrent pressure ulcers. A pressure ulcer can profoundly decrease functional independence. In addition, the financial burden to the health-care system can be extraordinary. The vigilance of clinicians is necessary to prevent pressure ulcers. Once an ulcer has formed, rational management strategies may hasten healing and decrease the incidence of complications.

Causation

Pressure ulcers are caused by both extrinsic and intrinsic factors. Extrinsic factors are the external conditions that contribute to ulcer formation, including excessive pressure, shearing, friction and maceration. Intrinsic factors are the conditions that are specific to the individual and include poor nutrition, spasticity, contractures, heterotopic ossification, recurrent urinary tract infection, urinary or fecal incontinence, impaired level of consciousness, substance abuse, and medication intake.

Pressure ulcers are most likely to occur over bony prominences. Common sites include the occiput, scapula, sacrum, ischial bursae, greater trochanter and heel. When tissue pressure exceeds capillary closing pressure, the result is progressive tissue ischemia with concomitant cellular death. The amount of tissue injury is related to the length of time and the amount of pressure the skin experiences.

Shearing forces between the skin and bone cause blood vessels to become angulated and stretched. Consequently, blood flow is compromised, which may result in tissue injury. Friction injury is similar to shearing, in that skin is abraded against the underlying bone and subcutaneous structures. In this case, however, cellular damage is the result of thermal injury. The last significant extrinsic factor is maceration, the softening of the skin secondary to moisture. Urinary incontinence, fecal soiling, and excessive perspiration can lead to maceration.

Prevention

Minimizing extrinsic factors (i.e., pressure, shear, maceration and friction) will decrease the incidence of pressure ulcers. If the patient is confined to bed, the entire skin surface must be assessed daily. To decrease pressure forces, the patient should be turned and positioned every two hours. Padding bony prominences may also be of value (e.g., "sheepskin boots" over heels or a pillow between legs when side-lying). During wheelchair sitting, patients, if capable, should engage in pressure relief strategies (e.g., wheelchair push up, shifting side to side, tilting or reclining of seating surface, etc.). Proper wheelchair fitting is critical to minimize pressure over seating areas (e.g., ischial bursae).

Shear and friction can be minimized by careful, skilled transfers. When a caregiver moves a patient in bed, care must be taken to avoid excessive shear forces. In SCI, spasticity may exacerbate shear forces and should be managed appropriately. Incontinence of feces and urine can be minimized by nursing and medical interventions.

Dressings For Pressure Ulcer Treatment
Table 1

Dressing Type	Comments
Coarse mesh gauze	As a dry dressing for minor abrasions; for wet-to-dry dressings; for wounds with scattered eschar or necrosis; as a topper dressing
Fine mesh gauze	For draining wounds or stomas; as a protective or topper dressing
Impregnated saline gauze (Mesalt)	For clean draining wounds
Impregnated charcoal gauze	For draining odoriferous wounds; as a cover dressing
Nonadherent pad (Alldress, Release, Telfa)	For clean wounds with scant draining, minor burns; as a cover dressing
Vaselinated gauze (Adaptic, Aquaphor, Vaseline gauze, Xeroform)	As a nonadherent dressing for minor to extensive burns
Polymeric membrane dressings (Bioclusive, Comfeel, Transparent, Opraflex, Opsite, Tegaderm)	For abrasions, Stage I or II pressure ulcers
Hydrocolloid dressing wafers (Comfeel products, Duoderm products, Replicare, Restore products)	For ulcers at Stage I through IV, vascular ulcers
Hydrogel dressings (Carrington Hydrogel Wound Dressing, Clear Site, IntraSite, Normigel, Nu-Gel)	For ulcers at Stages I through IV, for skin tears
Hydrocolloid and hydrogel flakes and pastes (Bard Absorption Dressing, Comfeel, DuoDerm, HydraGran, RepliCare)	For ulcers at Stages II and III, draining ulcers, vascular ulcers
Alginate sponges and ropes (Algosteril, Kaltostat products, Sorbsan)	For Stage II and III draining, vascular ulcers
Polymeric foam dressings (Allevyn products, Epi-Lock, Lyofoam products, Mitrafelx products)	For ulcers at Stages II through IV, venous ulcers, draining stomas and tubes

Editor's note: This list of products is not comprehensive, nor does products' listing constitute an endorsement by the editors or the publishers; the products serve only as examples. The comments in the "Indications" column of the table are generalized; please refer to specific manufacturer's instructions for each product's specific action and recommended use.

Indications

Is not indicated for weeping or open wounds because coarse mesh gauze will become entangled in granulating epithelium; for debriding only when used for wet-to-dry procedures

Is less likely to adhere to a draining wound

Is not recommended for dry wounds; uses fluid from the wound to produce a moist environment

Has activated charcoal embedded in dressing for odor control

Absorbs small amounts of drainage with minimal disruption of the wound bed; protects red granulating wounds

Is widely used for burns and abrasions; Xeroform has some antimicrobial properties

Provide a moist healing environment

Are available in various thicknesses; colloid interacts with fluid from the wound to provide a moist environment for wound healing and to promote epithelial migration; may allow for extended time periods between dressing changes; most are self-adhering to healthy tissue; may be contraindicated for infected ulcers

Three types: (a) self-adhering wafer type that has a low water content, can be changed up to once per week, and has small amount of absorption; (b) non-adhering wafer type that has a high percentage of water content and is usually changed daily; (c) a gel that is partially composed of water, has minimal absorption, and helps maintain a moist wound surface

Provide a moist environment; are effective for drainage control in deep, draining ulcers; can be used with gauze or other toppers to provide nonocclusive dressing with the benefits of a hydroactive dressing

Are highly absorbent for effective drainage control, provide a moist environment with low adherence; not indicated for wounds with scant drainage, as they can dessicate wound bed; might be contraindicated for infected wounds

Have high absorbency and low adherence; some are available with impregnated charcoal for odor control

Reprinted from McCourt A.E. (Ed.), *The Specialty Practice of Rehabilitation Nursing: A Core Curriculum* (3rd ed., p. 87), with permission of the Association of Rehabilitation Nurses, 4700 W. Lake Avenue, Glenview, IL 60025-1485. Copyright 1993.

Figure 9.1 **Staging of Pressure Ulcers**

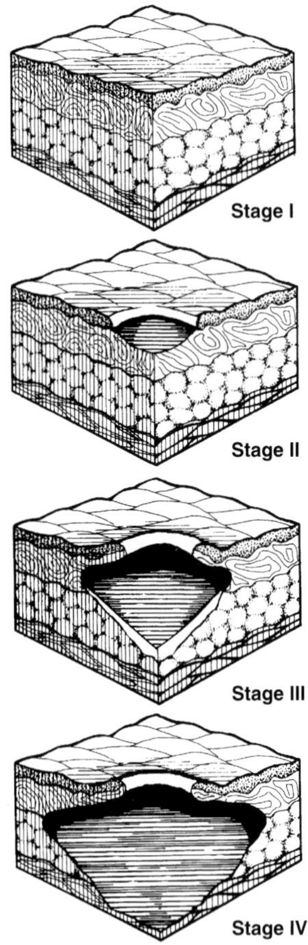

Stage I

Stage II

Stage III

Stage IV

Reproduced with permission from
National Pressure Ulcer Prevention Council.

Assessment

Proper documentation of clinical findings enables accurate assessment of improvement or worsening of a lesion. On occasion, a CT scan or MRI may assist in evaluating the depth and severity of a pressure ulcer. Healing or progression of the ulcer should be documented through objective assessment. Objective data include diameter of the ulcer, depth of the ulcer, tissue color, odor, and drainage color.

Stage I ulcers are characterized by non-blanching erythema of anatomically intact skin.

Stage II ulcers involve partial-thickness loss of skin, including the epidermis and, possibly, the dermis; the clinical presentation includes blisters, abrasions or shallow craters.

Stage III ulcers are characterized by destruction of the entire skin (epidermis and dermis). The injury progresses through the subcutaneous tissue.

Stage IV ulcers involve full-thickness skin loss with extensive destruction to the fascia, muscle, bone or joint. These ulcers may develop fistulas to the intestines, bladder or urethra.

Beds

Proper beds can aid in the prevention and treatment of pressure ulcers. There are several types of bed support surfaces. Static support surfaces, such as foam (Geo-Matt) or static air mattress (Waffle, Sof Care), are an appropriate choice for individuals who have reasonable bed mobility. At a minimum, a static support surface should have one inch of cushion between any bony prominence and the bed frame. Dynamic support surfaces (water, gel, alternating pressure pads), such as an overlay mattress, can be used with individuals who have impaired bed mobility and, therefore, are at high risk of pressure ulcers (e.g., a malnourished, unconscious C5 tetraplegic). These support surfaces are also appropriate for patients who have Stage I or II ulcers. This type of support surface may also be of value to those who unacceptably compress standard static support surfaces. Low-air-loss (Acucair, KinAir, PneuCare) and air-fluidized (Clinitron, FluidAir) beds may be indicated when a patient has already developed a large Stage III or IV pressure ulcer and has failed to improve with a dynamic overlay. These beds are also helpful for patients who have had a recent surgical flap procedure. Alternate support surfaces are expensive and should only be prescribed as a component of a comprehensive pressure ulcer management program.

Treatment

Every reasonable step should be taken to prevent pressure ulcers. Once a lesion has developed, however, rational treatment should be prescribed. To reduce the progression of the ulcer, the extrinsic factors that contributed to the formation of the ulcer should be identified and treated. In general, healing will be promoted if the wound remains clean, moist and debrided. A non-infected wound will also promote healing.

Management strategies for pressure ulcers can be divided into local and systemic therapies. Local therapies, which are delivered at the pressure ulcer site, include mechanical and chemical treatments. Mechanical methods include wound cleansing, debridement and dressing. Chemical interventions include creams and ointments. Systemic treatments include caloric and vitamin supplementation in addition to intravenous antibiotics.

A pressure ulcer should be cleansed on a regular basis. Normal saline is an excellent cleansing agent. Diluted iodine-based solutions (e.g., Provodine) have germicidal effects; theoretically, this agent impairs wound healing and is not recommended.

Debridement of necrotic tissue will promote wound healing and can be achieved by mechanical or chemical means. Debridement can be achieved by the use of a sharp instrument to remove the debris or devitalized tissue. Other mechanical methods include wet-to-dry gauze dressings, whirlpool therapy, wound irrigation, and dextranomers.

Autolytic debridement occurs when a synthetic dressing is used to cover the wound. This facilitates the natural enzymes produced by the skin to self-ingest the devitalized tissue. Collaginase compounds (e.g., Elase) are chemical debriding agents that can be applied to a wound. This method is contraindicated in infected wounds.

The ideal dressing for the pressure ulcer should keep the wound bed moist and the surrounding skin dry (Table 1). The dressing should control exudate and eliminate dead space. There are many commercially available dressings. However, there is little evidence to support the superiority of any particular brand. As such, the choice of dressings is partly determined by the experiences and preferences of the practitioner. The table on pages 60 and 61 provides some guidelines for selecting dressings.

If an ulcer is not healing and there is a clinical suspicion of wound infection (i.e., foul odor, purulent drainage, extensive marginal erythema), then a trial of topical antibiotics for a period of two weeks may be considered. Topical antibiotics are not indicated if the patient has sepsis or osteomyelitis. The topical agent should treat the putative pathologic organism. Examples of frequently used topical treatments are silver sulfadiazine, triple antibiotic (neomycin, polymyxin B and bacitracin), and metronidazole cream. Wound cultures are of questionable value, as they may reflect colonization and not the putative pathological organism. Topical antibiotics are available in ointments and creams. Ointments are non-water soluble and should be used with caution because they may impair wound drainage. If a wound appears infected on clinical grounds, and has not responded to topical antibiotics, a trial of systemic antibiotics may be considered.

Hospitalization and intravenous antibiotics are indicated for complications such as sepsis, advancing cellulitis or osteomyelitis. Osteomyelitis is sometimes difficult to diagnose. Bone biopsy is the "gold standard" for diagnosis. Abnormalities may also be recognized on MRI and plain X-rays. Furthermore, the erythrocyte sedimentation rate and white blood cell (WBC) counts may be elevated. The proper management of osteomyelitis requires the involvement of plastic surgery, orthopedic surgery, and infectious disease services. Long-term intravenous antibiotics and possible surgical debridement may be required.

The healing of any wound requires adequate calories, proteins and vitamins. Malnourished individuals should receive dietary supplements (e.g., Ensure, Sustical). Vitamin C, vitamin A and zinc supplementation may assist with wound healing (Table 2). A nutritionist can formulate an acceptable dietary plan. Caloric intake should be based on ideal body weight (IBW), which is calculated by the following formula:

IBW for males = 50 kg + [2.3 x (height in inches - 60)]
IBW for females = 45.5 kg + [2.3 x (height in inches - 60)]

Stage III and IV ulcers may require surgical treatment. A number of surgical procedures are available, including direct closure, skin grafts, skin flaps, and musculocutaneous flaps. The general medical condition of the patient, as well as the extent of the ulcer, will guide the treatment team. Surgical success is enhanced by ensuring adequate nutrition, treating spasticity, smoking cessation, and control of wound and urinary tract infections prior to surgery. Post-operative care requires a supervised "seating protocol" after a minimum of two weeks of bed rest. Tolerance to pressure is promoted by slowly increasing sitting time, while closely assessing the surgical site for erythema that does not resolve within 10 minutes of pressure relief. Patient education programs for pressure ulcer prevention are essential to long-term success.

Strategies To Prevent Pressure Ulcers

- Vigilant daily skin surveillance
- Turn and position every two hours
- Minimize friction, shear and moisture
- Pad bony prominences
- Encourage early safe mobilization
- Optimize nutrition

Treatment of Pressure Ulcers

- Identify and accurately stage ulcers
- Minimize pressure time, shear, moisture, friction
- Consider alternative bed surface
- Optimize caloric and protein intake
- Zinc, vitamin C, vitamin A supplementation
- Cleanse wound regularly
- Gentle debridement
- Treat infection
- Dressings should be moist and fill empty space
- Skin around wound should be dry
- Surgical consultation for Stage III and IV ulcers

Table 2
Nutritional Interventions For Pressure Ulcer Management

Intervention	Rationale	Dose
protein	necessary for collagen synthesis	1.25 -1.5 gram/kg per day of IBW
calories	aids in tissue defense and wound repair	31 - 34 calories/kg per day of IBW
iron	required for oxygen transport cofactor for collagen synthesis	ferrous sulfate 300 mg tid or ferrous gluconate 650 mg tid
zinc oxide	cofactor for collagen synthesis	25 - 50 mg qd
vitamin C	aids in collagen synthesis	500 - 1000 mg qd
vitamin A	for stimulation of epithelial tissue	20,000 - 25,000 IU qd

Suggested Readings

Bergstron N, Bennett MA, Carlson CE, et. al. Treatment of pressure ulcers. Clinical Practice Guidelines, Number 15; Rockville, MD: U.S. Department of Health and Human Services; 1994 December.

Dituno J, Formal C. Chronic spinal cord injury. New England Journal of Medicine 1994; 330:550-556.

Kraft CF. Skin care. Topics in Spinal Cord Injury Rehabilitation 1996; 2(1).

Krasner D. Chronic wound care 1991; Pennsylvania: Health Management Publications; 1991.

Chapter 10

Contracture Management

Steven Nussbaum, MD

Pathology

Contractures are defined as a fixed loss of passive joint range of movement secondary to pathology of connective tissue, tendons, ligaments, muscles, joint capsules or cartilage. Traumatic, inflammatory, ischemic or infectious factors can cause collagen proliferation. These collagen fibers may initially be deposited in a disorganized manner. If the joint is taken through full functional range (either actively or passively), the newly-deposited collagen will organize in a linear fashion. Alternatively, if the joint is immobilized, the collagen matrix will organize in a tightly packed manner, and a contracture will result.

Classification

Contractures can be classified as arthrogenic, soft tissue or myogenic. Arthrogenic contractures are caused by pathology involving the intrinsic joint components. Examples include cartilage damage secondary to osteoarthritis, or joint incongruency as the result of an intra-articular fracture. Arthrogenic contractures generally cause range of movement restrictions in multiple directions.

Soft tissue contractures result in the shortening of tendons, ligaments and skin. These contractures generally cause restriction of movement in one direction.

Myogenic contractures can be divided into intrinsic and extrinsic lesions. Intrinsic muscle contractures are secondary to a primary disorder of muscle fibers. An example would be muscular dystrophy in which histologically abnormal muscle is present. Most traumatic SCI patients suffer from extrinsic muscle contractures as the result of muscles being placed in a shortened position for extended periods of time. The muscle, however, is histologically normal. Factors that can lead to extrinsic contractures include spasticity, immobility, improper positioning and pain. Heterotopic ossification can also cause extrinsic myogenic contractures.

Common Locations of Contractures

In the lower extremities, ankle plantarflexion, hip flexion, and knee flexion contractures are common. In the upper extremities, elbow flexion and supination contractures are possible, depending on the level of injury. Some patients also may develop shoulder adduction and internal rotation contractures. Muscles that cross multiple joints, such as the biceps, hamstrings, tensor fascia lata, and gastrocnemius, are predisposed to contracture formation.

Beneficial Contractures

Some contractures may improve functional status and thus should be encouraged to develop. For example, C6 tetraplegics have intact wrist extension. This allows the utilization of the tenodesis effect in which active movement of one joint results in the passive movement of other joints. In C6 tetraplegia, the active extension of the wrist (due to an intact extensor carpi radialis) causes passive flexion of the MCP, PIP and DIP joints. Shortening of the paralyzed flexor digitorum profundus and superficialis will facilitate this passive flexion. This results in a type of prehension that will increase functional independence. To achieve this tenodesis effect, the MCP, PIP and DIP joints must be allowed to contract in slight flexion (approximately 20 degrees). A wrist-driven hinge orthosis (e.g., the RIC or TIRR Orthosis), which stabilizes the thumb, index finger and middle finger, will further promote tenodesis. A biceps flexion contracture may also be useful. When an individual has poor biceps strength, a slight elbow flexion contracture may improve the mechanical advantage of the muscle.

Prevention of Disadvantageous Contractures

Contractures can be prevented with early mobilization, range of movement exercises, proper positioning, and orthotic devices. Contracture prevention requires the coordinated effort of the medical, nursing and therapy services. Patients must be encouraged to get out of bed as soon as practical. The therapeutic exercise program must be tailored to the patient's level of injury. If the patient is capable, ambulation with devices should be encouraged. Patient and caregiver education emphasizing the importance of performing a home stretching program is essential.

Splinting is an effective adjunctive treatment for contracture management. It is not, however, a substitute for a comprehensive rehabilitation treatment program. Orthotic devices can be prescribed to maintain positioning of the hands, elbows, knees and ankles. Patient comfort is essential for a successful splinting program. Skin irritation and pain can result in non-compliance. After initial fabrication of the orthosis, the patient should be monitored every 30 minutes for problems with skin tolerance. If pressure areas are not detected, a two-hour wearing schedule is initiated. The patient may increase the wearing schedule to a full night as skin tolerance allows.

Improper bed positioning may contribute to contractures. The supine position encourages hip flexion and ankle plantarflexion contractures. Placing a pillow under a patient's knees will encourage hip and knee flexion contractures. Another bed position to avoid is one that encourages extreme adduction and internal rotation of the shoulder. Proper bed positioning can minimize contracture formation. Patients should be advised to lie prone in bed to minimize hip flexion contractures. When in bed, the shoulder should be placed in abduction and some external rotation. This can be achieved with strategic placement of pillows. The progression of ankle flexion contractures can be prevented with ankle foot orthosis. Flexion and supination contractures at the elbow can be prevented with resting night splints or bivalved casts, both of which promote elbow extension and pronation.

Proper wheelchair seating and positioning is also essential in preventing the formation of contractures. Contractures and subluxation of the shoulder can be prevented with the placement of armrests and lapboards on the wheelchair. Forward placement of the armrest encourages extension of the elbow.

The pelvis should be maintained with a slight anterior tilt, thus encouraging normal lordosis in the lumbar spine and kyphosis in the thoracic spine. A posterior pelvic tilt will encourage kyphosis of the lumbar spine, causing the head and neck to lean forward. Extensions, also called hip blocks, placed on a wheelchair laterally keep the pelvis symmetrical and help to align the lower extremities. A short hip block stabilizes the pelvis while a long hip block prevents excessive abduction. Leg straps can be used to prevent adduction of the lower extremities while sitting in the wheelchair. Footrest height can be adjusted to change the position of the ankle, knee and hip. The trunk can be stabilized by utilizing laterally placed trunk supports and by modifying the seat to recline 10 degrees.

Treatment of Contractures

Every reasonable step should be taken to prevent contractures. Once a contracture has formed, however, a variety of interventions are available. The factors that are contributing to contracture formation, such as pain, spasticity, inflammation and improper positioning, should be treated. Treatments can be divided into three groups: physical, medical and surgical.

Physical interventions include therapeutic heat (i.e., ultrasound) prior to a stretching program. A terminal sustained stretch is essential. Caution must be used with therapeutic heat in areas with impaired sensation. Regional osteoporosis may also have caused fragile bones, and vigorous stretching may lead to a fracture.

Serial casting or dynamic splinting can be an adjunctive therapy to a stretching program. Serial casting (Figure 10.1) utilizes a plaster cast that is applied to a limb that has been pre-stretched approximately five degrees. The cast is subsequently removed in three to five days, and a new cast is placed after the limb is stretched another five to 10 degrees. This process continues until the contracture has been reduced. Serial casting should be discontinued if pain or pressure ulcers develop. Dynamic splinting utilizes splints with movable parts to counter contracting forces. Dynasplints and outrigger splints are examples of dynamic splints.

In refractory cases, orthopedic surgical procedures, such as joint manipulation, tendon release, and tendon lengthening, can be considered. If pain or spasticity are contributing to contractures, these conditions should be managed appropriately. These topics are discussed in other chapters of this monograph.

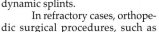

Figure 10.1 **Serial Casting**

Suggested Readings

Yarkony GM. Contractures complicating spinal cord injury: incidence and comparison between spinal cord center and general hospital acute care. Paraplegia 1985; 23:265-271.

Halar E, Bell K. Contracture and other deleterious effects of immobility. In: DeLisa J, editor: rehabilitation medicine principles and practice. Philadelphia: Williams & Wilkins; 1988; 448-455.

Hill J, Presperin J. Deforming control. In: Intagliata S, editor. Spinal cord injury — a guide to functional outcomes in occupational therapy. Rockville, MD: Aspen; 1986; 49-81.

Chapter 11

Autonomic Dysfunction

Nancy DeSantis, DO

SCI compromises the motor, sensory and autonomic pathways. Impairment of the motor tracts leads to weakness, whereas impairment of the sensory tracts leads to dysesthesias and anesthesia. Dysfunction of the autonomic pathways is associated with the clinical findings of autonomic dysreflexia such as severe hypertension and headaches. Persons with SCI, however, may have other dysautonomic features such as baseline hypotension, orthostatic hypotension, impaired thermoregulation, and diminished sweating.

Cardiovascular Function

Blood pressure is the product of cardiac output and total peripheral resistance. Cardiac output is the product of heart rate and stroke volume. Stroke volume is directly related to cardiac venous return. Heart rate and blood pressure are influenced by the effects of the sympathetic and parasympathetic nervous system. In SCI, the parasympa-

Table 1
Medications to Treat Hypotension in SCI

Generic Name	Brand Name	Initial Dose	Maximum Dose	Mechanism	Precautions
fludrocortisone acetate	Florinef	0.1 mg	0.4 mg	mineralocorticoid that promotes sodium and water retention	hypertension CHF hypokalemic alkalosis peripheral edema hypernatremia
ephedrine sulfate	Ephedrine	25 mg bid	50 mg tid	alpha and beta agonist	tachycardia arrhythmias palpitations headache urinary retention insomnia sweating tremulousness
midodrine hcl	ProAmatine	2.5 mg tid	10 mg tid	alpha-1 agonist	headache paresthesias dysuria puritis piloerection

thetic vagus fibers, which originate in the brain stem, are usually spared. However, the sympathetic fibers, which originate in the thoracic and lumbar spinal cord, may be disrupted by SCI, depending on the level of injury.

Hypotension

Hypotension can present in the acute and/or chronic phase of SCI. Hypotension is related to decreased vascular tone, diminished circulating catecholamines, and impaired venous return. An orthostatic component is frequently identified. It is not unusual for patients to have sitting systolic blood pressures in the 60 mm Hg - 80 mm Hg range. Some individuals experience dizziness and syncope, whereas others are asymptomatic. Symptoms may be exacerbated by meals, as blood is shunted to the gastrointestinal system for digestion. Treatments include thigh high compression stockings and abdominal binders. Caregivers should slowly sit persons with SCI from the recumbent position. If these strategies are unsuccessful, fludrocortisone, ephedrine and midodrine can be considered.

Table 2
Medications to Treat Chronic Dysreflexia

Medication	Brand Name	Initial Dose	Maximum Dose	Mechanism	Precautions
phenoxybenzamine	Dibenzyline	10 mg bid	40 mg tid	alpha antagonist	avoid alcohol postural hypotension tachycardia nasal congestion miosis
clonidine (oral) or clonidine (weekly patch)	Catapres Catapres TTS	0.1 mg qd 0.1 mg/24 h	0.8 mg tid 0.3 mg /24 h	central acting alpha-2 agonist	orthostatic hypotension withdrawal hypertension sedation constipation dry mouth weakness skin rash pruritus tricyclics may decrease effectiveness
terazosin	Hytrin	1mg qhs	10 mg bid	alpha-1 antagonist	hypotension sedation headaches fatigue syncope
prazosin	Minipress	1 mg bid	5 mg tid	alpha-1 antagonist	hypotension sedation headache fatigue syncope

Impaired Thermoregulation

Maintenance of normal body temperature requires an intact autonomic and neuroendocrine system. Thermoregulation is coordinated by the hypothalamus. When core body temperature is decreased, homeostatic mechanisms cause shivering. In addition, blood flow to the extremities is reduced. When core body temperature is elevated, the normal homeostatic response is to increase sweating and to shunt blood toward the extremities. In SCI, these normal regulatory mechanisms may be dysfunctional due to compromised autonomic pathways. Hyperthermia and hypothermia are commonly seen in persons with SCI. Prior to concluding that a patient has hyperthermia (i.e., quad fever) secondary to dysautonomia, other causes of fever should be excluded. Sometimes, hyperthermia and hypothermia may be secondary to ambient temperature (poikilothermia) and may be corrected by adjusting the thermostat. Individuals with impaired thermoregulation should have homes and vans that have excellent climate control systems.

Autonomic Dysreflexia

Autonomic dysreflexia (AD) is a syndrome characterized by a sudden rise in systolic and diastolic blood pressure in response to noxious stimuli below the level of injury. It is most often associated with bradycardia. However, tachycardia and other cardiac rhythm disturbances are possible. Other symptoms include sweating or flushing above the level of the injury, pallor below the level of injury, sudden pounding bilateral headache, nasal congestion, anxiety, and, rarely, visual disturbances. Typically, AD is associated with injuries at or above the T6 level; however, there are cases reported with lower thoracic lesions. The elevations in blood pressure may range from 20 mm Hg (systolic and/or diastolic) above the baseline to in excess of 200 mm Hg systolic and 100 mm Hg diastolic. Untreated AD can lead to intracerebral hemorrhage and death.

Autonomic dysreflexia occurs after the period of spinal shock has resolved. Individuals must have an intact spinal cord below the level of injury to develop AD. Noxious stimuli below the neurological level travel into the spinal cord and cause reflex sympathetic constriction of the vascular structures. This may result in increased preload and resultant hypertension. The elevated blood pressure is detected by the carotid baroreceptors, which results in increased vagal tone. This usually results in bradycardia. However, heart rate is influenced by the opposing effects of the sympathetic and parasympathetic systems. As such, tachycardia is also possible. In uninjured persons, this reflex vascular constriction is modulated by higher brain stem, subcortical and cortical centers. This modulation, however, is absent or impaired in persons with SCI.

Table 3
Common Causes of Autonomic Dysreflexia

Bladder distention	Kidney stones	Cholecystitis	Restricting
Fecal impaction	Bladder stones	Ingrown toenails	clothing
Urinary tract	Skin ulcers	Bone fractures	Cystoscopy
infection	Epididymitis		Gastric ulcers

To manage autonomic dysreflexia, the precipitating cause must be identified and treated. The individual should be placed in the sitting position in order to induce venous pooling and decrease preload. Blood pressure should be monitored every five minutes. If the systolic blood pressure is above 150 mm Hg and the precipitant cause cannot be readily treated, medical therapy should be instituted. Topical or sublingual nitrates are appropriate choices. Topical nitroglycerin has a rapid onset and should be applied above the level of the lesion. If hypotension results, the nitropaste should be wiped away, and the individual should be placed in a recumbent position and the legs elevated. If dysreflexia cannot be controlled, admission to an intensive care unit for intravenous nitroglycerin or nitroprusside should be considered. Nifedipine sublingual should not be used as it has been associated with stroke. Oral nifedipine, however, can be considered.

Chronic Autonomic Dysreflexia

Chronic autonomic dysreflexia develops in some individuals. Successful management requires the recognition and treatment of precipitating conditions (i.e., bladder spasticity, pressure ulcers, etc.). There are a number of medications that may be utilized to manage chronic autonomic dysreflexia (Table 2). However, medications may also lower baseline blood pressure and contribute to orthostatic hypotension.

Suggested Readings

Banister R, Mathias C, editors. Autonomic failure: A textbook of clinical disorders of the autonomic nervous system. Third edition. Oxford University Press; 1992; 839-881.

Braddom RL and Rocco JF. Autonomic Dysreflexia: A survey of current treatment. American Journal of Physical Medicine and Rehabilitation 1991; 70:234-241.

Colachis SC, III. Autonomic hyperreflexia with spinal cord injury. Journal of the American Paraplegia Society 1992; 15:171-186.

Erickson RP. Autonomic hyperreflexia: pathophysiology and medical management. Archives of Physical Medicine and Rehabilitation 1980; 610:431-440.

Consortium for Spinal Cord Medicine. Acute management of autonomic dysreflexia: adults with spinal cord injury presenting to healthcare facilities. Clinical Practice Guidelines. Spinal Cord Medicine 1997 February.

Chapter 12

Upper Motor Neuron Syndrome and Spasticity

Mark Kaplan, MD

The upper motor neuron syndrome consists of positive and negative findings. Positive manifestations include spasticity, athetosis, primitive reflexes, rigidity and dystonia. Negative findings include weakness, paralysis and fatigue.

Spasticity, an abnormality of muscle tone, becomes clinically apparent as spinal shock resolves. It is characterized by a velocity-dependent resistance to passive joint movement. Other clinical findings include hyperactive muscle stretch reflexes and clonus. Many persons with SCI also experience flexor and cutaneo-motor spasms. Although these abnormalities of motor control are not considered manifestations of spasticity, they may respond to many of the same management strategies. In the chronic phase of SCI, an increase in spasticity or spasms may be secondary to medical complications such as urinary tract infection, bowel impaction or syrinx.

Measuring Spasticity

The Ashworth and Modified Ashworth Scales are the most commonly used scoring instruments and are based on findings during clinical examination. The Spasm Frequency Score is based on the reporting of the individual experiencing abnormalities in muscle tone. Researchers use electrophysiological parameters, such as F-wave and H-reflex measurements (threshold, latency, amplitude, etc.), to quantify spasticity. However, changes in electrophysiological measures may not correlate with clinical or functional improvements. Some studies have utilized the pendulum test, as well. This test involves placing the examinee in a supine position with the legs hanging over the edge of the plinth. The leg is allowed to fall, and knee movement is assessed with an electrogoniometer.

Modified Ashworth Scale

0 = No increase in muscle tone

1 = Slight increase in muscle tone, manifested as a catch-and-release or by minimal resistance at the end of range of motion

1+ = Slight increase in muscle tone, manifested by catch, followed by minimal resistance throughout the remainder (less than half) of the range of motion

2 = More marked increase in muscle tone through most of the range of motion, but the affected part is easily moved

3 = Considerable increase in muscle tone; passive movement difficult

4 = Affected part(s) rigid

Spasm Frequency Score

0 = No spasms
1 = Mild spasm induced by stimulation
2 = Infrequent, full spasm occurring less than once per hour
3 = Spasms occurring more than once per hour
4 = Ten or more spasms per hour, or continuous contraction

Contracture and Spasticity

Many times, contracture and spasticity coexist in SCI. Increased tone leads to diminished movement. The result is a cycle that, if untreated, can have deleterious consequences.

Upper Motor Neuron Syndrome and Function

Not all the manifestations of the upper motor neuron syndrome require treatment. Sometimes, spasticity and spasms can be beneficial. For example, a patient may use knee extensor spasticity to assist in transferring from a sitting to standing position. Spasticity of knee extensors may also increase stability during the stance phase of gait. Spasms may be used to assist with bed mobility. Alternatively, increased muscle tone can be deleterious. For example, spasticity may contribute to a poor seating position, which could contribute to contractures and skin breakdown. Flexor spasms of the lower extremity may cause a person with SCI to strike a limb against the leg rests of a wheelchair.

Indications for Treatment of Spasticity

Decrease pain	Minimize contractures	Improve seating
Improve nursing care	Assist in prevention and	Improve gait and transfers
Improve hygiene	healing of pressure ulcers	Improve self-care activities

Areas of Skin Breakdown Associated With Spasticity

Muscle Group	Area of Potential Skin Breakdown
Shoulder adductors	Axilla
Elbow flexors	Antecubital fossa
Finger flexors	Palm
Hip adductors	Perineum
Knee flexors	Sacrum, heels

Pain and Spasticity

Spasticity may produce pain directly or due to the prolonged contraction of a muscle. Contractures and pressure ulcers can cause pain, which may increase nociceptive afferent impulses and lead to further spasticity.

Treating Spasticity

The treatments for spasticity include physical, medical and surgical interventions. The first step in treating spasticity is to recognize and manage stimuli that may be contributing to increased tone such as urinary tract infections, bladder stones, fecal impaction, heterotopic ossification, or pressure ulcers.

Positioning

Tone may be affected by head and body positions. The tonic neck and vestibular reflexes may be useful in modulating spasticity. For example, some persons with SCI have diminished tone in the partially recumbent position. As such, this position is incorporated into wheelchair-sitting strategies. Casting or splinting an extremity may also diminish spasticity.

Table 1
Anti-Spasticity Medications

Medication	tizanidine	clonidine	dantrolene sodium	diazepam	baclofen
Brand Name	Zanaflex	Catapres (oral) Catapres TTS (weekly patch)	Dantrium	Valium	Lioresal
Mechanism of Action	alpha-2 agonist (centrally acting)	alpha-2 agonist (centrally acting)	Inhibits Ca2+ release	GABA facilitation	GABA analogue
Starting Dose	2 mg bid	0.1 mg PO bid 0.1 mg/24-hour patch	25 mg qd	2.5 mg bid	2.5 mg bid
Maximum Dose*	36 mg/day	2.4 mg/day 0.3 mg/24-hour patch	400 mg/day	60 mg/day	80 mg/day
Montly Cost Range** Brand name	$15.47 – $245.46	$39.79 – $285.48 $26.28 – $80.73	$25.74 – $172.48	$12.94 – $270.89	$11.58– $128.63
Generic	no generic	$12.98 – $91.70 no generic patch	no generic	$4.45 – $41.64	$7.79 – $70.79
Common Side Effects	drowsiness weakness dry mouth mild hypotension	weakness sedation constipation skin rash dry mouth pruritus orthostatic hypotension withdrawal hypertension	weakness sedation dizziness parasthesia nausea diarrhea hepatitis	sedation weakness depression ataxia memory loss dependence	sedation fatigue weakness nausea dizziness parasthesia decreased seizure threshold hallucinations and seizures if withdrawn abruptly

Table adapted from Whyte J, Robinson KM. Pharmacologic management. In: Glenn MB, Hyte J, editors. The practical management of spasticity in children and adults. Malvern, PA: Lea and Febinger; 1990: 222.

*Manfacturers' recommended maximum dose. Some clinicians prescribe higher doses.

**Ranging from initial to maximum dose. Source: Boston Medical Center Outpatient Pharmacy.

Modalities

Cryotherapy and electrical stimulation can reduce spasticity for several hours after application. Sustained cold over a muscle group (i.e., 20 minutes) may decrease spasticity. Alternatively, quick cooling or electrical stimulation of an antagonist of a spastic muscle group may result in reciprocal inhibition and thereby decrease muscle tone. Many individuals with SCI, however, are insensate below their neurological level, and modalities must be prescribed with extreme caution.

Stretching

A stretching program can minimize tone. It should be incorporated into the individual's daily routine. When stretching muscles, a terminal sustained stretch is essential for diminishing tone. The benefit of stretching may last throughout the day.

Medications

Side effects of medications may limit their use (Table 1). The most commonly used first-line agent is baclofen. However, some experts believe that tizanidine is a more appropriate choice. The annual cost of therapy (medications, required laboratory tests, repeat physician visits, etc.) should be considered in treatment decisions.

Nerve Blocks

Nerve blocks involve injecting a medication close to a nerve causing temporary or permanent dysfunction (Figure 12.1). A temporary nerve block can be completed with lidocaine or bupivocaine. This may allow a clinician to evaluate the potential benefits of a nerve block and facilitate the use of other interventions such as serial casting or dynamic splinting. To perform a longer acting nerve block (chemical neurolysis) agents such as phenol and ethanol may be employed.

Nerve blocks can be performed at any anatomically accessible nerve. It is possible to block nerve fibers at the root, plexus or peripheral nerve. Some muscle groups (e.g., iliopsoas) cannot be practically blocked at a distal site, so the neurolysis must be completed at the nerve root.

Nerve blocks completed on sensorimotor nerves can result in unwanted dysthesias and, rarely, anesthesia. However, if the person with SCI is insensate at the site of the nerve block, the potential sensory side effects are less of a concern. Reducing sensory input, however, may be beneficial, as nociceptive inputs sometimes exacerbate spasticity. A motor branch block is a type of chemical neurolysis in which the most distal motor branches of a peripheral nerve are blocked. Motor branch blocks require more needle insertions and can be tedious to perform. There is, however, a lower risk of sensory complications. Other complications from nerve blocks include weakness and sensitivity to the injected agent. Phenol blocks can lead to fibrosis of the nerve and make future nerve blocks at the same site more difficult.

Paravertebral nerve root blocks have more potential side effects. If during a lumbar paravertebral block, the subarachnoid space is inadvertently compromised, incontinence, sexual dysfunction and ascending paralysis are possible.

The duration of effect from chemical neurolysis is variable. On average, the effects of the procedure should last between three and nine months. However, in some individuals, the benefits persist for many years. Nerve blocks should be used as part of a comprehensive rehabilitation treatment program; by adding a stretching program, the benefits may be prolonged.

Localization of the nerve is critical for a successful nerve block. The closer the medication is delivered to the nerve, the less medication is required and fewer side effects are likely. The site of injection can be localized with a variable intensity pulse stimulator.

A needle coated with teflon (except at the tip) is attached to a syringe. Current is delivered through the needle by a stimulator. As the needle approaches the nerve, a muscle contraction will be elicited. The closer the needle is to the nerve, the less current will be required. With this technique, the medication can be delivered very close to the nerve.

Nerve blocks are commonly performed on muscles innervated by the median, ulnar, obturator, sciatic and tibial nerves. In general, blocking a motor branch is preferred to a mixed sensorimotor nerve.

Botulinum Toxin

Botulinum toxin is a neuromuscular blocking agent that inhibits the effects of acetylcholine. Botox injection, unlike a nerve block, does not require the use of a stimulator. However,

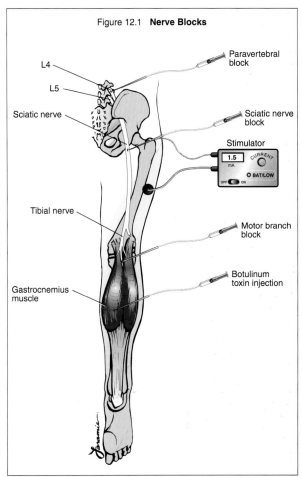

Figure 12.1 **Nerve Blocks**

L4
L5
Sciatic nerve
Paravertebral block
Sciatic nerve block
Stimulator
1.5 mA
CURRENT
BAT/LOW
OFF ON
Tibial nerve
Motor branch block
Botulinum toxin injection
Gastrocnemius muscle

some clinicians use EMG signals to assist in muscle localization. Risks of injection include reaction to the injectant, bleeding and infection. This procedure has a duration of effect from one to six months and may be more appropriate for patients soon after injury. The onset of effect typically occurs several days after injection and the maximum effect is obtained over a period of several weeks. This may be of benefit in allowing patients to gradually adapt to their new muscle strength. Disadvantages include the high cost relative to anesthetic or phenol injection. Subsequent injections may become less effective due to antibody mediated resistance to the botulinum toxin.

Baclofen Pump

Intrathecal baclofen delivery may be effective in patients whose spasticity is not controlled by other means. A temporary catheter is placed into the intrathecal space and a 50 microgram test dose of baclofen is given. A 100 microgram dose can be tried if the lower dose is ineffective and there are no significant side effects. If effective, a permanent catheter is implanted. The pump with a reservoir is placed subcutaneously and refilled at one- to three-month intervals. Potential side effects include infection, catheter breakage, drowsiness, hypotension and weakness. With an overdose, respiratory depression is possible. Autonomic dysreflexia can be precipitated if the intrathecal baclofen is abruptly discontinued.

Surgical Treatment

Destructive neurosurgical procedures, such as rhizotomy and cordotomy, are rarely performed. Orthopedic procedures can also be considered in selected cases. Irreversible procedures should not be performed until neurological recovery has plateaued, typically up to one year post-injury.

Suggested Readings

Bohannan, RW. Smith, MB. Interrater reliability of a Modified Ashworth Scale of muscle spasticity. Physical Therapy 1987; 67:206-207.

Priebe MM, Sherwood AM, Thornby JL, Kharas NF, Markowsky J. Assessment of spasticity in spinal cord injury with a multidimensional problem. Archives of Physical Medicine and Rehabilitation 1996; 77: 713-716.

Kaplan M. Tizanidine: Another tool in the management of spasticity. Journal of Head Trauma Rehabilitation 1997; 12(5):93-97.

Glenn MB, Whyte J, editors. The practical management of spasticity in children and adults. Malvern, PA: Lea and Febinger; 1990.

Stein AB, Pomerantz F, Schechtman J. Evaluation and management of spasticity in spinal cord injury. Topics in Spinal Cord Injury Rehabilitation 1997; 2(4):70-83.

Chapter 13

Heterotopic Ossification

Douglas E.Garland, MD

The term heterotopic ossification (HO) is preferred to such terms as ectopic ossification, paraosteoarthropathy, or myositis ossificans when discussing the formation of new bone near joints as a consequence of SCI. Heterotopic refers to the occurrence in more than one area. Microscopically, the bone is a true "ossific" process, progressing de novo to new bone formation rather than to calcification of soft tissue.

Genetics and Patient Predisposition

Strong support for some type of genetic predisposition to HO formation is derived from reseach into the hereditary disorder fibrodysplasia ossificans progressiva (FOP). This disorder is inherited as an autosomal dominant trait with full penetrance and variable expression. It is a disorder of connective tissue, with skeletal malformations and HO. The natural history of HO associated with FOP has similarities to the natural history of HO from other causes, especially neurogenic HO.

The association of human leukocyte antigens (HLA) with neurogenic HO has been documented. An increased prevalence of HLA-B18 and HLA-B27 antigens has been reported in some SCI patients with HO. However, follow-up studies from other centers have not confirmed these findings. This system cannot presently predict susceptibility to HO.

Clinical Presentation

Clinically significant HO (i.e., resulting in significant limitation in joint range) affects approximately 10 percent to 20 percent of SCI patients. Ankylosis occurs in fewer than 10 percent of these lesions. Symptoms of HO are usually recognized within the first two months post-injury. It is unusual for HO to be diagnosed beyond six months post-SCI. HO usually presents in the paralyzed extremities (i.e., below the neurological level).

Clinical findings include erythema, pain and swelling. Other manifestations include decreased joint range of movement, increased spasticity, and low-grade fevers. With incomplete lesions, patients may experience pain. Differential diagnosis includes deep venous thrombosis, cellulitis, abscess, septic joint, hematoma and tumor.

The most common sites for HO in SCI patients are the hips and knees. In the hip, the lesion is usually anterior to the hip joint. It courses in a plane from the anterior iliac spine toward the lesser trochanter. Pseudoarthrosis, which allows for passive movement, is commonly noted. Although HO may occur anywhere in the anterior thigh, it is most commonly noted in the distal anteromedial knee. Ankylosis is uncommon. HO rarely involves the shoulder or elbow. In such cases, the mass is usually small and can be noted in any plane. Other sites are rare.

Diagnosis

Elevated levels of serum alkaline phosphatase (SAP) are associated with clinically significant HO. This is particularly true at the hip. SAP levels begin to rise to the upper limits of normal within the first two weeks of injury. At three weeks, the SAP levels may exceed normal values, and the elevation may persist for up to five months. The SAP level parallels the clinical course of HO.

The three-phase radionuclide bone scan is the best method for early detection and confirmation of HO. This test requires an intravenous injection of 99mTc-labeled methylene diphosphonate. The radioisotope concentrates in areas of increased bone activity. The three phases of a bone scan are the dynamic blood flow phase (nuclear angiogram), immediate static phase (blood pool phase), and the delayed static phase. Abnormalities in the first two phases of the bone scan will be present prior to abnormalities in the third phase. Clinicians should insist on a three-phase study, and not a single static phase study. A three-phase bone scan can detect HO as early as two to three weeks after the onset of the lesion.

Radiographs may provide confirmatory evidence of HO. Although plain films may detect HO as early as three weeks after injury, radiographic detection may not be confirmatory until two months after the initial clinical presentation.

The precise role of computed tomography (CT) scanning as a clinical tool for diagnosis and a measure of maturation of HO is not established. CT scanning clearly defines HO and its relationship to muscles, vessels and nerves. This study should be considered prior to surgical excision.

Treatment

The clinical significance of HO varies from patient to patient, and management decisions must be individualized. In some individuals, the HO is of little functional significance and requires no intervention. Others suffer from multiple lesions that impair function significantly. The majority of patients can be satisfactorily managed with physical therapy and medications.

Physical Therapy

Physical therapy can be helpful in the management of HO. The goal is to maintain functional range of movement. The affected joints should be gently moved through functional range. Vigorous force, however, should not be used, as this may lead to further ectopic bone formation.

Medical Management

Prophylactic HO treatment with medications for every SCI is probably not warranted. If there is a clinical suspicion of HO, then a bone scan is appropriate.

Patients diagnosed with HO can be treated with etidronate disodium (EHDP). This medication is a structural analog of inorganic phosphate and limits ossification by blocking the formation of hydroxyapatite crystals. The oral dose is 20 mg/kg per day, and may be given in one dose or in two divided doses for a period of up to six months. Some clinicians recommend that initial treatment should be with intravenous EHDP (300 mg per day) for the first three days, followed by oral therapy. The most common side effects of EHDP are nausea, vomiting and diarrhea. In studies with dogs, pathologic fractures have developed after nine months of treatment.

Nonsteroidal anti-inflammatory drugs (NSAID) have not been studied extensively in HO associated with SCI. They may eventually be proven effective, but presently are adjuncts to EHDP. NSAID may be indicated subsequent to surgical resection. Indomethacin is the preferred NSAID, at 25 mg tid. Alternate choices are ibuprofen 300-400 mg tid and aspirin 650 mg tid.

Surgery

Surgery is appropriate in selected cases that are refractory to conservative management. Surgical indications include functionally impaired joint mobility, impaired sitting, and significant spasticity. Surgical treatment may range from a wedge resection to the complete removal of the lesion. The goal is not to eradicate the ectopic bone, but rather to allow for functional range of movement. Surgery should be planned when the HO is at a quiescent state (i.e., normal SAP levels, mature radiographic appearance, and baseline bone scan). It may be take up to 18 months for a lesion to reach this inactive stage. Postoperative prophylaxis is necessary. Combination therapy is desirable. Radiation at 600 - 750 rads in single or divided doses is appropriate. As well, EHDP or NSAID are necessary for a period of three to six months.

Suggested Readings

Bonovac K and Gonzalez F. Evaluation and management of heterotopic ossification in patients with spinal cord injury. Spinal Cord 1997; 35:158-162.

Garland DE. A clinical perspective of common forms of acquired heterotopic ossification. Clinical Orthopedics 1991; 263:13-29.

Garland DE and Orwin JF. Resection of heterotopic ossification in patients with spinal cord injuries. Clinical Orthopedics 1989; 242:169.

Garland DE, Rubayi SS, Harway EC, Pompan DC. Proximal femoral resection and vastus lateralis flap in the treatment of heterotopic ossification in patients with spinal cord injury. Contemporary Orthopedics 1995; 31:341.

Orzel JA, Rudd TG. Heterotopic bone formation: clinical, laboratory, and imaging correlation. Journal of Nuclear Medicine 1985; 26:125-132.

Chapter 14

Psychological Adaptation

J. Scott Richards, PhD

Psychological Function During Acute Rehabilitation Admission

During the first few weeks to months following SCI, the whole continuum of human emotional responses and defenses against what could be overwhelming reality can be seen. The older rehabilitation literature describes stage theories for this process, which imply a predictable if not necessary sequence of emotional and cognitive reactions as persons with SCI move toward "adjustment." There is, however, no universal path to adjustment. Adjustment is not an end point but a lifelong process of adaptation. However, there are a number of commonly experienced emotional reactions. Often, these reactions become clinically appreciated in the rehabilitation setting, when the individual with SCI initially confronts his limitations.

Depressive behavior is often present. It can be difficult to distinguish between an acceptable reactive depressive episode (i.e., grief secondary to loss of function) as opposed to a problematic major depression. Persistent sadness (dysphoria) in response to the recognition of functional losses is common, appropriate and typically time-limited. Support, encouragement and empathic listening are all helpful responses to this process when it occurs. Deciding when someone has a major depression, however, can be more problematic. Clinical signs of depression, such as sleep disturbance, weight loss, loss of appetite, diminished energy, and diminished interest in sexual functioning, can all be sequelae of medical complications and not directly reflective of a major depressive episode.

Anxiety is often evident as well and, in a smaller proportion of cases, full-blown post-traumatic stress disorder can be seen. Judicious use of anxiolytics can be helpful as a short-term intervention, but needs to be weighed against the implicit message that adjustment to injury can best be done passively through medications rather than actively through coping. If anxiety impairs the learning that is required to participate in the rehabilitation program, then medication should be considered. Behavioral treatment approaches for anxiety should also be considered, including relaxation training and imagery deconditioning techniques.

Other reactions, such as anger, hostility and withdrawal, are often seen as well. However, staff members are often baffled by the lack of apparent negative emotional reactions in some persons with SCI. There is no convincing evidence that the absence of strong negative emotions bodes poorly for the future. Patients need to be assessed carefully to ascertain their true level of psychological distress.

Whether to confront the patient directly with the permanence of his injury is an issue that must be decided without the benefit of empirical data. The clinical consensus seems to be that physicians should directly respond to the patient's questions with regard to prognosis. If the patient has not requested prognostic information about neurological recovery, it is potentially harmful to the therapeutic relationship to directly confront the individual.

Cognitive Concerns

Given the epidemiology of SCI, with a large percentage of injuries caused by rapid deceleration events (e.g., motor vehicle crashes), there should be a high index of suspicion for concomitant traumatic brain injury. This will be obvious in some cases in terms of impaired memory, judgment, impulse control and reasoning, but may be much more subtle and more difficult to detect in others. Concomitant significant traumatic brain injury may compound the length of time required to learn new tasks and may impact other aspects of rehabilitation such as social and familial adjustment. In the more severe cases, in which lingering cognitive and behavioral deficits persist, return to school and work, as well as successful social integration, can be compromised.

The clinician should also be alert to pre-injury conditions or characteristics that compromise current cognitive functioning, including prolonged substance abuse histories, prior traumatic brain injury, learning disabilities, or genetic disorders. Since the success of rehabilitation depends largely on new learning, this is an important issue.

Personality and Behavioral Issues

Most SCI individuals do not fit the "norm" in terms of psychological epidemiology. The best predictor of future behavior is still past behavior. Hence, deriving a careful history with regard to developmental, legal, psychiatric, vocational and social difficulties is most important. A disproportionate percentage of the events that cause SCI are associated with the use or misuse of legal and illegal substances. Return to substance abuse in the rehabilitation unit is usually prevented or limited by the milieu, but research suggests a high return to substance abuse post-discharge and is an issue worthy of follow up and monitoring.

Personality testing, as well as a good behavioral history, can provide excellent prognostic information about the likelihood of compliance short- and long-term with regimens that can prevent secondary complications. This kind of behavioral "red flag" is not necessarily limited to those with a clear substance abuse history.

Long-Term Issues

Many times, a parent or spouse (often a mother or wife) becomes a permanent caregiver. The individual with SCI often experiences markedly decreasing emotional distress over the first year post-injury; the caregivers, in contrast, may have markedly increased distress. This occurs as the caregivers' support system dwindles and the amount of help provided by others diminishes. Promoting respite care (formal or informal) and attending to the emotional and physical health of the caregiver is important.

Suicide, as a cause of death, is higher among persons with SCI when compared to their age-matched able-bodied counterparts. Active suicide gestures or attempts rarely occur during the acute rehabilitation admission, but are more likely to occur later as a function of lack of recovery, interpersonal difficulties, financial distress, and significant affective disorders. Substance abuse can also be a "trigger" for suicide, particularly when accompanied by diminished social support and meaningful activity on a day-to-day basis. Suicide gestures and threats need to be taken seriously and responded to with appropriate referral to ensure safety and adequate treatment.

Many persons with SCI do not return to paid employment. The financial benefits of disability are often of sufficient magnitude to act as a disincentive to return to paid employment. For example, many individuals would lose medical benefits and reimbursement for personal care assistants if they engaged in remunerative employment. If the patient is amenable, vocational evaluations and training options should be pursued vigorously. In the absence of a desire to attempt a return to competitive employment, persons with SCI should be encouraged to pursue meaningful activities such as wheelchair sports, family activity, church work, or other avocational pursuits.

Chronic pain is an issue for a significant minority of persons with SCI. The etiology of the discomfort may be musculoskeletal or neurological, and a thorough evaluation is appropriate. However, in many cases, no clear anatomical disorder can be established, and the patient may be diagnosed with an undifferentiated chronic pain syndrome. Pain can be an avenue for medication seeking, particularly with those who have a substance abuse or prescription drug use history. Depression or anxiety can magnify the extent and impact of chronic pain. The optimal management of chronic pain requires a multidisciplinary approach. Active versus passive coping methods should also be pursued.

Role of the Psychologist

The psychologist can provide systematically derived information of help to the patient, family and staff via structured interviews and formal psychological testing. Some psychologists use a standard battery of psychological tests. Others use combinations of interviews and tests, depending on the particular referral question and problem. It is helpful to provide specific referral information to help the psychologist guide the assessment. It is also helpful to consider a standing referral order to the psychologist for all new persons with SCI. This helps destigmatize the referral process (i.e., all SCI patients are evaluated by the rehabilitation psychologist). Psychological assessment at the earliest stages of injury (i.e., ICU) may be therapeutic. Interaction with the patient during initial rehabilitation admission also facilitates contact post-discharge. It is at this juncture where family and patient coping mechanisms become most taxed.

Psychologists can provide information about personality, intellect, affect, mood, and cognition. Identifying strengths and weaknesses in these areas is essential for vocational reintegration, as well as financial and driving competency. This information can be used to guide treatment decisions and discharge plans. Assessment of problematic pre-injury behaviors, which are likely to be predictive of future difficulties, can also be accomplished. Psychological evaluation can be useful in formulating behavioral management strategies.

Psychologists participate in educational activities for persons with SCI. Educationally focused groups tend to work better than traditional group psychotherapy. Topics commonly discussed include sexuality, body image changes, disability rights, assertiveness, and family relations. Individual interventions can also be provided, ranging from stress management techniques, such as relaxation training and biofeedback, to cognitive-behavioral approaches stressing improvements in problem solving ability and coping style. Behavioral programming is sometimes necessary and can be quite effective and helpful in managing problem behaviors. This requires the cooperation of the entire staff and is an activity that requires a considerable investment of time and resources. Sex education and counseling are important interventions, which are discussed in the next chapter. Psychologists often facilitate and coordinate peer visitation programs to assist individuals with SCI in the coping process. Timing for this intervention is critical as peer visitation is unlikely to be beneficial if the person with SCI is not receptive to the idea.

SCI has a demonstrated negative impact on romantic relationships. Physicians need to recognize developing and ongoing stressors, as well as behavioral and emotional difficulties in persons with SCI post-discharge. If marital or family difficulties are identified, the psychologist can provide expert assessment. If further counseling or therapy is required, the psychologist can organize treatment. Alternatively, care may be coordinated with other mental health professionals.

Suggested Reading

Consortium for Spinal Cord Medicine. Depression following spinal cord injury: A clinical practice guideline for primary care physicians. Paralyzed Veterans of America, 1998.

Dijkers, MP, Buda Abela M, Gans BM, Gordon WA. The aftermath of spinal cord injury. In: Stover SL, DeLisa JA, Whiteneck GG, editors. Spinal cord injury: clinical outcomes from the model systems. Gaithersburg, MD: Aspen Press; 1995; 185-212.

Richards JS, Kewman DG, and Pierce CA. Spinal cord injury rehabilitation. In Elliott TE, Frank R, editors. Handbook of rehabilitation psychology; APA Press; 1988; 68-82.

Rohe DE. Psychological aspects of rehabilitation. In: DeLisa JA, editor: Rehabilitation Medicine: Principles and Practice. Philadelphia: J.B. Lippincott; 1988, 68-82.

Treischmann, RB, Spinal cord injuries: Psychological, social and vocational rehabilitation. 2nd edition. New York: Demos Publications; 1988.

Chapter 15

Sexuality and Spinal Cord Injury

Stanley Ducharme, PhD

Introduction

With longer life expectancies following SCI, the emphasis in rehabilitation over the past decade has gradually shifted to improving quality of life. Toward this goal, issues related to sexuality must be addressed by the rehabilitation team in both the acute and chronic stages of SCI. Providing sexual education to patients and their partners is best accomplished by an interdisciplinary team approach in which both medical and psychological issues can be addressed.

Male Sexual Act

Erectile and ejaculatory function are complex physiological activities that require the interaction between the vascular, nervous and endocrine systems. Erections are controlled by the parasympathetic nervous system, whereas ejaculation is controlled by the sympathetic nervous system.

In the simplest of terms, erection is controlled by a reflex arc that is mediated in the sacral spinal cord. A reflex involves an afferent and efferent limb. The afferent limb consists of somatic afferent fibers from the genital region that travel through the pudendal nerve into the sacral spinal cord. The efferent limb involves parasympathetic fibers that originate in the sacral spinal cord. These fibers travel through the cauda equina and exit via the S2 to S4 nerve roots. The post-ganglionic parasympathetic fibers secrete nitric oxide, which causes relaxation of the smooth muscle of the corpus cavernosum and increases blood flow to the penile arteries. Consequently, the vascular sinusoids of the penis become engorged with blood, and the result is an erection. This reflex is modulated by higher brain stem, subcortical and cortical centers. In addition, erectile function is influenced by hormonal factors such as testosterone.

Ejaculation signals the culmination of the male sexual act and is primarily controlled by the sympathetic nervous system. Similar to the sympathetic innervation of the bladder, these fibers originate in the thoraco-lumbar spinal cord and travel into the sympathetic chain. These fascicles then travel through the splanchnic nerves into the hypogastric plexus. After synapsing in the inferior mesenteric ganglion, postganglionic fibers travel through the hypogastric nerves to supply the vas deferens, seminal vesicles and ejaculatory ducts in the prostate.

Female Sexual Act

The physiology of the female sexual act has not been studied as well as the male sexual act. However, female sexual satisfaction is dependent on a complex interaction of the endocrine and nervous systems. Sexual excitation is the result of psychogenic and physical stimulation. This arousal is manifested by vaginal lubrication and tightening of the introitus. Stimulation of the genital region, including the clitoris, labia majora, and labia minora, causes afferent signals to travel via the pudendal nerve into the S2 to S4 segments of the spinal cord. These fibers interact with efferent parasympathetic fibers that project through the pelvic nerve. The result is dilation of arteries to perineal muscles and tightening of the introitus. In addition, the parasympathetic fibers cause the Bartholin's glands to secrete mucus, which aids in vaginal lubrication.

Female orgasm is characterized by the rhythmic contraction of the pelvic structures. Female orgasm also results in cervical dilation, which may aid in sperm transport and fertility.

Sexual History

A simplified sexual history should be part of the initial clinical assessment. Key elements include physical capabilities, past sexual activities, and current sexual function. In addition, the clinician should inquire into partner availability, partner satisfaction, sexual orientation, behavioral repertoire, and past sexual abuse. Open-ended questions will facilitate better communication. Topics of a more sensitive nature should be reserved for later in the interview, when a therapeutic relationship has been established.

Psychological Considerations

Adaptation to an SCI is a gradual process that extends over a prolonged period of time. Successful sexual adjustment is influenced by many factors such as age at time of injury, quality of social supports, physical health, gender, and severity of the injury. Losses need to be mourned so that the remaining strengths can be nurtured and developed. To achieve satisfying sexual adjustment, a person with an SCI will have to learn to value their new sexual abilities, as opposed to recapturing the past.

After a traumatic injury, individuals typically go through a period of reduced sexual drive. Although libido is not affected by SCI, it may be diminished by depression, trauma of the injury, or medications. Initially after injury some persons with SCI may deny the importance of sexual issues. Other individuals may be reluctant to discuss issues related to sexuality due to cultural or personal reasons. Other patients may go through a period of sexual "acting out" (i.e., unacceptable sexually explicit language, inappropriate unwanted physical contact with staff, etc.) while on the rehabilitation unit.

During the acute rehabilitation phase, a sensitive discussion regarding sexuality is appropriate. The person with SCI may inquire about issues such as dating, attractiveness, relationships, parenthood and physical appearance. Other topics of interest many include erections, lubrication, sensation, orgasm, ejaculation and fertility. Many individuals will inquire about sexuality as it relates to bladder and bowel function. Even if the patient does not initiate discussion about these topics, it is important for members of the rehabilitation team to provide basic information.

Male and Female Arousal

Men and women with SCI often lack sensation at traditional erogenous areas such as the genitals and nipples. As such, stimulating these areas may result in penile erections or vaginal lubrication, but not necessarily sexual pleasure. However, other areas, sometimes not normally recognized as erogenous areas, such as the ears, eyelids and neck, can be stimulated to provide sexual arousal. Some individuals find the skin surfaces around the neurological level to have heightened tactile sexual response.

Male Sexual Funtion: Erections, Ejaculation and Orgasm

Men with SCI may obtain reflexogenic or psychogenic erections. Reflex erections are secondary to manual stimulation of the genital region. Psychogenic erections are the result of erotic stimuli that result in cortical modulation of the sacral reflex arc. In general, erections are more likely with incomplete injuries (both upper and lower motor neuron), than complete injuries. Many times, men with SCI can only maintain an erection while the penis is stimulated, and the quality of the erection is insufficient for sexual satisfaction. As such, the erection must be augmented with devices, medications or a penile implant for satisfactory sexual function.

In men with SCI, the ability to ejaculate is less common than the ability to obtain an erection. The rate of ejaculation varies depending on the location and nature of the neurological injury. In complete upper motor neuron lesions, the ejaculation rate is estimated at 2 percent. In incomplete upper motor neuron lesions, the ejaculation rate is estimated to be somewhat higher at 32 percent. Many men who are able to ejaculate experience retrograde ejaculation into the bladder; some may experience dribbling of semen.

The experience of orgasm in men with SCI is variable. Some individuals describe a primarily emotional event. Others experience generalized muscle relaxation or a pleasurable sensation in the pelvis or at the sensory level. Other men report orgasm to be nonexistent following the injury.

Oral Therapy for Male Sexual Dysfunction

Sildenafil (Viagra) was approved by the FDA in 1998, and may have a significant role in the treatment of erectile dysfunction for men with SCI. Sildenafil is a type 5 phosphodiesterase inhibitor that prevents the intracorporal breakdown of cyclic GNP. It is rapidly absorbed after oral administration and is taken approximately 60 minutes before anticipated sexual activity. It is most effective for men who are capable of achieving reflex erections. It can assist the man in gaining further rigidity and in sustaining the erection for penetration. Sildenafil is contraindicated in men taking nitrates due to the risk of profound hypotension. Many men with SCI have low baseline blood pressures, and this agent should be prescribed with caution. In addition, this drug is not recommended for those individuals with cardiac disease. Side effects noted in the otherwise well population include facial flushing, dyspepsia, headache and visual disturbances.

Intracavernosal Injection Therapy

Therapy with intracavernosal injection (Figure 15.1) of papaverine, alprostadil, and phenotolamine is an accepted treatment of erectile dysfunction. Initiating this therapy necessitates a referral to a urologist. Initially, individuals are given small doses of the pharmacological agent, and the dose is increased until a satisfactory erection is obtained for intercourse. Sometimes, a mixture of agents is prescribed. Erections should not persist beyond four hours. Many tetraplegics have impaired hand function and will require a cooperative partner to perform the injection. In some cases, a commercially marketed penile autoinjector can be easier to manipulate. Priapism is a possibility; therefore, both partners should be properly trained. Some individuals with incomplete injuries may experience pain at the injection site. Penile fibrosis is also a potential risk of intracavernosal therapy.

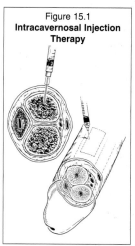

Figure 15.1
Intracavernosal Injection Therapy

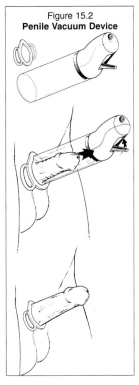

Figure 15.2
Penile Vacuum Device

Transurethral Therapy

Recently, transurethral delivery systems for administering agents that result in erections have been approved. The medication delivered is usually alprostadil. This treatment is generally not as effective as intracavernosal therapy. Many men are not satisfied with the rigidity of the erections obtained.

Penile Vacuum Devices

These devices create a vacuum around the penis (Figure 15.2). As a result, blood is drawn into the corporal spaces. A band is then slipped off the plastic cylinder around the base of the penis to maintain penile tumescence. Ejaculation may be retarded due to the constriction of the urethra. However, newer models are available with constricting bands that are less likely to diminish ejaculation.

Vacuum devices are non-invasive, economical and efficacious. However, these devices require some degree of manual dexterity For many men with tetraplegia, the partner must be willing to assist with the procedure. In addition, men must transfer out of the wheelchair and be in a recumbent position to obtain a good vacuum seal at the base of the penis. Individuals with incomplete injuries may experience pain, discoloration, and coldness at the penis. Constriction rings should not remain in place for more than 30 minutes. Longer time periods may be associated with potential skin breakdown. Vacuum devices are more accepted by men in more established sexual relationships. Some men use vacuum devices to augment erections obtained with oral medications. Vacuum devices are commonly used in underdeveloped nations where pharmacotherapy is unavailable or not affordable.

Penile Implants

Penile implants are considered when other treatments have been unsuccessful, especially if trauma has disrupted the penile vascular system. It also may be indicated if severe Peyronie's disease is a factor. Implants are not considered in the first year post-injury so that persons with SCI can make emotional adaptations to the injury and explore less invasive options for sexual activity. There are a number of different devices, ranging from the simple malleable prosthesis to more complex hydraulic prostheses. Generally, the choice of prosthesis is related to individual preference and financial constraints.

Figure 15.3 **Penile Vibroejaculator**

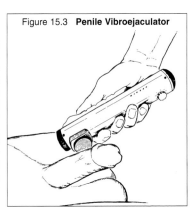

Male Fertility

The ability to father a child correlates with the frequency of ejaculation. Successful pregnancy rates range from 10 percent to 35 percent. In general, men with incomplete lesions (both upper and lower motor neuron) are more likely to become fathers than are those with complete lesions. Conditions that may contribute to infertility include retrograde ejaculation, repeated urinary tract infections, and altered testicular temperature. Newer methods of obtaining semen samples include rectal electroejaculation or penile vibroejaculation (Figure 15.3). Both of these techniques may precipitate autonomic dysreflexia.

Female Sexual Function: Sexual Arousal and Vaginal Lubrication

Most women with SCI can achieve some level of vaginal lubrication. This lubrication can be mediated by reflexogenic or psychogenic factors. Individuals with incomplete (both upper and lower motor neuron) injuries are more likely to have satisfactory lubrication. If vaginal lubrication is unsatisfactory, then a water soluble lubricant can be recommended. Sildenafil may be of value in women with SCI by increasing blood flow to the perineum, and increasing vaginal lubrication, which may improve sexual satisfaction. However, there are no controlled studies on the female SCI population.

Female Fertility

Immediately after injury, 44 percent to 58 percent of women suffer from temporary amennorhea. Menstruation usually returns within six months post-injury. Neither the level nor the completeness of the injury appear to be associated with interruption of menstrual cycles. In a small percentage of women with SCI, there are also changes in cycle length, duration of flow, amount of flow, and amount of menstrual pain. Most women with SCI are fertile.

Birth Control

The issue of birth control can be somewhat problematic for women with SCI. Condoms provide contraception, as well as diminish the risk of transmission of sexually transmitted diseases. A diaphragm may be another acceptable option if the individual has adequate hand dexterity or a cooperative partner. Oral contraception is associated with increased incidence of thromboembolism, and must be prescribed with caution in women with SCI. Oral contraceptives that contain only progesterone may be safer than medications that contain both estrogen and progesterone. IUD may be associated with increased incidence of pelvic inflammatory disease. Untreated PID may lead to autonomic dyssreflexia. In addition, women with SCI may not be able to perceive if the device has migrated out of the cervix.

Pregnancy

Pregnant women with SCI have an increased risk of urinary tract infections, leg edema, autonomic dysreflexia, constipation, thromboembolism and premature birth. Since uterine innervation arises from the T10 to T12 levels, patients with lesions above T10 may not be able to perceive uterine contractions or fetal movements. It may be difficult to differentiate between pregnancy induced hypertension (pre-eclampsia) and autonomic dysreflexia. Autonomic dysreflexia may be the only clinical manifestation of labor. During the second and third trimester, pregnant women may have difficulties in performing functional tasks that were previously completed independently. Transfers may require the assistance of a caregiver, and a power wheelchair may be necessary for mobility. Locating an obstetrician and anesthesiologist with a supportive attitude, an accessible office, and experience in SCI can be difficult in many areas.

Urinary and Fecal Incontinence

Urinary and fecal incontinence at inopportune times and subsequent social rejection are major fears of some people with SCI. A bladder or bowel accident may occur at any time during courtship, sexual activity, or during social events. The embarrassment, shame, and humiliation associated with incontinence create undue anxiety and are often regarded as a major reason for social isolation or the termination of a relationship.

To minimize untimely episodes of incontinence, the bladder should be emptied prior to sexual activity. Foley catheters, if present, can be taped to the side of the penis with a condom placed over the catheter. Females can engage in sexual intercourse despite the presence of a Foley catheter by taping the catheter to the abdomen. Despite the best management program, sexual stimulation can cause urinary and/or fecal incontinence. Embarrassing passage of gas from the vagina, bowel or ostomy bag can be avoided by gentle thrusting, coital positioning, and a careful diet. Fluids should be limited during the hours preceding sexual activity. Towels should be available to manage episodes of urinary or fecal incontinence.

Conclusion

Sexual adaptation after an SCI is a gradual process that involves psychological and physical adjustments. The availability of new medications, devices and procedures have greatly enhanced the possibility of having a satisfactory sexual life after an SCI. Toward this end, the rehabilitation team has a responsibility to provide sexual information and counseling during the acute and chronic stages of SCI.

Suggested Readings

Boller F, Frank E. Sexual dysfunction in neurological disorders. New York: Raven Press; 1982.

Ducharme, S, Gill, K. Sexuality after spinal cord injury. Baltimore, MD: Paul Brooks Publishing Co.; 1997.

Leyson, J. Sexual rehabilitation of the spinal cord injured patient. Clifton, NJ: Humana Press; 1991.

Sipski, M, Alexander, C. Sexual function in people with disability and chronic illness. Gaithersburg, MD: Aspen Publication; 1997.

Chapter 16

Aging and Spinal Cord Injury

Elizabeth Roaf, MD

Introduction

The care of patients with long-term SCI is a challenging and rewarding task. Optimal care of this population requires an understanding of both the rehabilitation and medical issues. Of equal importance is an appreciation of the physiology of aging. People with chronic SCI suffer from many of the same medical disorders as able-bodied individuals. The clinical manifestations of these medical conditions, however, may be atypical (e.g., age of onset, signs and symptoms) due to the complex physiologic changes associated with SCI. Therefore, every person with an SCI should have a skilled primary care physician; this practitioner may be an internist, physiatrist or family physician.

The Aging Lung

Prior to considering the effects of chronic SCI on lung function, the effects of aging must be understood. Vital capacity (total exhalation after a maximal inspiration) normally peaks at approximately age 20, then gradually diminishes by 1 percent per year. Although vital capacity decreases with age, total lung capacity does not. Thus, the residual volume of the lung increases as the vital capacity diminishes. The loss of vital capacity may occur due to lack of deep-breathing activities as older adults frequently become more sedentary. Vital capacity also diminishes acutely with lung infections and mucus plugging. Patients with baseline reduced vital capacities and tidal volumes who do not take occasional deep breaths can rapidly develop collapse of the small airways and alveoli (microatelectasis). In addition, the elastic recoil of the lung diminishes with aging. Microatelectasis, with concomitant diminished lung capacity, may result in non-uniform ventilation, especially in the dependent portions of the lung.

Cough may be weakened due to age-related changes in lung mechanics, as well as decreased intercostal and abdominal muscle strength. Weakened cough impacts secretion clearance and may prolong the course of respiratory infections.

Pulmonary Processes in Chronic SCI

Pulmonary diseases are major sources of morbidity and mortality in SCI. By some estimates, respiratory illnesses (i.e., pneumonia and bronchitis) are the leading cause of mortality in long-term SCI patients. Tetraplegics and high-level paraplegics have impaired cough mechanisms due to paralysis of the abdominal and intercostal muscles. These patients have difficulty clearing secretions and are at high risk for pneumonia.

Treatment of an SCI patient with an acute respiratory infection includes the standard approach to individuals with respiratory disease (i.e., history, physical examination, complete blood count, blood cultures, chest X-ray, sputum analysis, antibiotics, etc.). Loosening of secretions should be attempted with warm mist via tracheostomy mask or half face mask. Nebulizer treatment with albuterol may be needed. Inhaled, oral or intravenous steroids may be indicated. As SCI patients have impaired pulmonary mechanics, intubation may be required.

Beyond these standard approaches, individuals with chronic SCI may need aggressive physical therapy interventions, including frequent suctioning, chest percussion, postural drainage, and assisted cough ("quad cough"). These treatments can be provided by the respiratory or physical therapy services. The frequency of these interventions should be individualized, but, in some cases, therapy is required every two hours. Oxygen saturation should be monitored frequently, and arterial blood gas (ABG) measurement should be done in patients with a known history of carbon dioxide retention or those who appear to be fatiguing.

If ventilation appears to be a necessary intervention, noninvasive positive pressure ventilation should be considered. Generally administered by a mask that fits over the nose, noninvasive positive pressure ventilation may be either continuous (CPAP) or bilevel (BIPAP). Although these methods are generally used for chronic hypoventilation syndromes, short periods of CPAP and aggressive secretion management may prevent intubation in an acute crisis. This should be considered in individuals with high-level lesions in which extubation may be challenging.

Individuals with long-term disability have often had multiple different courses of antibiotics and may have strains of bacteria that are highly resistant to many antibiotics. Patients with tracheostomies may be colonized with pseudomonas, which can make analysis of sputum (colonization vs. infection) complex. Infectious disease consultation may be warranted in such cases.

Global Alveolar Hypoventilation

Global alveolar hypoventilation (GAH) is an insidious, restrictive process that may compromise pulmonary function in SCI patients. GAH is an ongoing, subclinical loss of ventilatory function due to loss of pulmonary compliance from chronic hypoventilation or scarring. This condition can lead to progressive respiratory failure and subsequent need for long-term ventilation. Chronically, it may be exacerbated by obesity, kyphosis and scoliosis. Subclinical hypercapnia and sleep disorders may also exacerbate GAH. Symptoms of worsening restrictive lung disease include nightmares, morning headaches, daytime drowsiness, dyspnea on exertion, orthopnea, and generalized fatigue. Caregivers may note paradoxical breathing.

Assessment of lung function should be a part of routine health-care maintenance, especially in those patients with complete high cervical lesions. Surveillance of lung function should include periodic arterial blood gas measurement to assess the degree, if any, of carbon dioxide retention. In addition to arterial blood gas monitoring, pulmonary function testing should be ordered every few years in tetraplegic individuals and some at-risk high-level paraplegics.

Chronic ventilation may become necessary to sustain life in some individuals who develop chronic hypoventilation. Ventilation may be invasive or noninvasive. The most common types of noninvasive positive pressure ventilation used are CPAP and BIPAP, which are often administered nasally via mask. Alternatives to CPAP and BIPAP include intermittent positive pressure ventilation (IPPV) via mouthpiece and negative pressure ventilators (e.g., raincoat, cuirass and mini iron lung). IPPV may initially be prescribed for episodic use throughout the day to maintain adequate carbon dioxide exchange. The raincoat ventilation device covers the thorax and has long sleeves that allow for a tight seal to the body. The cuirass ventilator is a hard shell-shaped device that fits over the chest. A tube (similar in appearance to a vacuum cleaner hose) is connected to the device which causes negative pressure and facilitates ventilation. The mini iron lung is a more compact version of the iron lung used in the past to treat polio. Successful negative pressure ventilation requires a small body habitus without significant kyphosis and scoliosis.

Cardiac Disorders

Coronary heart disease is the leading cause of death in adults in the United States. As life expectancy of individuals with SCI has increased, mortality from coronary artery disease has increased. Risk factors include elevated total serum cholesterol, increased low-density lipoprotein, depressed high-density lipoprotein, obesity, family history of heart disease, diabetes, smoking, hypertension and immobility. More recently fibringen levels, homocystinemia and uric acid levels have been noted to have roles in the development of coronary artery disease. Individuals with SCI may be at increased risk for CAD due to relative inactivity, insulin insensitivity or diminished HDL levels. The wide variations in blood pressure from autonomic instability secondary to SCI may cause intimal damage.

In tetraplegia and high-level paraplegia, pain perception is impaired due to disruption of spinal afferent pathways from the heart and coronary vessels. This disruption is less profound in incomplete lesions. Nociception may be further impaired by coexisting medical conditions (e.g., diabetes with autonomic neuropathy). Cardiac ischemia and infarctions may present with unusual pain referral patterns, symptoms of autonomic dysreflexia, or other atypical presentations. Silent ischemia and infarction are also a possibility.

Screening for heart disease begins with a thorough clinical assessment. Risk factors should be identified. However, physical exam findings must be interpreted with caution. For example, chronic peripheral edema may be due to dependency and lack of muscle tone, and not secondary to right heart failure. Auscultation of the lungs may reveal crackles that may be secondary to left heart failure. Alternatively, these findings may be secondary to pulmonary scarring and atelectasis.

Investigations to evaluate ischemic heart disease may include arm ergometry exercise testing in paraplegics or low-level tetraplegics. Persantine thallium or MIBI studies may also be helpful. Since standard cardiac stress tests are not as diagnostically valuable in women, a dolbutamine echocardiography should be considered. This test is also useful in those individuals who cannot perform upper arm ergometry.

In SCI patients, echocardiography may show atrophy of cardiac musculature in a symmetric fashion. The symmetrical atrophy is most likely due to lack of cardiac loading from immobility, profound orthostatic hypotension, and diminished venous return. These echocardiographic abnormalities are different from the concentric cardiac hypertrophy seen in able-bodied patients with hypertension.

SCI patients with CAD should be managed in similar fashion to other patients. Modifiable risk factors should be addressed. The spectrum of interventions available to able-bodied patients should be offered to SCI patients (i.e., lifestyle changes, medications, angioplasty and CABG).

Introduction of medications should be done cautiously as many patients with SCI have low baseline blood pressures and, consequently, may not be able to tolerate traditional doses of anti-anginal medications.

Osteoporosis

Osteoporosis is a group of disorders affecting bone, characterized by decreased osteoblastic formation relative to osteoclastic resorption. This results in a net loss of bone. Osteoporosis may be generalized or localized.

Following an acute SCI, patients suffer from regional osteoporosis syndrome. Twenty to 50 percent of bone mass in lower extremities is lost within the first few months. Bone mobilization may occur beginning as early as the first two weeks following injury. More typically, bone resorption begins around week four to five post-injury. Peak mobilization is at approximately the 16th week post-injury. The mobilization of calcium gradually diminishes and reaches a plateau between five to 24 months post-injury. This is due to both increased osteoclastic activity post-injury and decreased osteoblastic activity. Most patients will experience hypercalciuria and hydroxyprolinuria.

Some male patients with acute cervical lesions may develop clinically significant hypercalcemia secondary to osteoporosis. Symptoms of hypercalcemia may include nausea, vomiting, malaise, anorexia, headache, gastric distention, abdominal pain, fecal impaction and depression. With severe hypercalcemia, seizures, cardiac arrhythmia and death are possible. Treatment of hypercalcemia begins with hydration with normal saline solution followed by diuresis with furosemide. Treatment bisphosphonates (etidronate, alendronate) may be needed in refractory cases. If the hypercalcemia is severe (symptoms of cardiac or CNS impairment) management should be in an intensive care unit.

Osteoporosis is defined as bone density less than or equal to 2.5 standard deviations from the mean on bone densitometry evaluation. Laboratory evaluation of osteoporosis should include measurement of serum calcium (to rule out bony metastases), phosphorus, parathormone (PTH, elevated in hyperparathyroidism), and serum alkaline phosphotase. Serum levels of calcium, phosphorus, alkaline phosphatase and PTH should be normal in individuals with osteoporosis. Individuals with SCI should be screened yearly for hyperthyroidism (TSH, T4 levels) since this is a treatable cause of osteoporosis.

There is an increased risk of fractures from profound disuse osteoporosis in SCI. Paraplegics will develop osteoporosis in the lower extremities. Quadriplegics also develop osteoporosis in the distal upper extremities. However, SCI is not associated with osteoporosis in the spine. Osteoporotic fractures may occur as early as a few years post-injury. The risk of osteoporosis may be lower in individuals with significant spasticity in their limbs; moderate to severe spastic muscles may exert forces on bone and decrease bone resorption.

Femur fractures are commonly encountered osteoporotic fractures in long-term SCI patients. They may occur subsequent to significant trauma such as a fall. However, minor trauma associated with transfers or PROM exercises may precipitate a fracture. This condition may present with pain, increased spasticity, swelling, erythema, autonomic dysreflexia or even low-grade fevers. With any fracture, orthopedic consultation is essential. Many times, femur fractures in SCI patients are managed non-operatively. Malunion and nonunion should be avoided. Malunion can lead to impaired sitting. As a result, patients may develop pressure ulcers and contractures. Impaired sitting can also lead to pelvic obliquity and scoliosis.

Slowing the progression of osteoporosis is essential. Although the literature is replete with information regarding interventions for prevention and treatment in the otherwise healthy population, the literature on safe, appropriate, effective treatment of osteoporosis for individuals with SCI is inadequate. Supplementation with vitamin D (400 to 800 international units daily) is recommended. Calcium supplementation is controversial in persons with SCI due to the increased risk of developing kidney and bladder stones. In individuals with long-term SCI, screening bone densitometry may be indicated. In selected patients, a trial of a bisphosphonate (Fosamax) or calcitonin, in addition to vitamin D, should be considered.

Musculoskeletal Pain

The incidence of chronic pain in the SCI population is estimated between 20 percent and 50 percent. Pain may be musculoskeletal, neuropathic or visceral in origin.

Upper extremity pain is common. People with SCI load joints that do not normally bear weight (i.e., shoulder, elbow and wrist). This predisposes them to painful upper extremity conditions. Symptoms of upper extremity pain, dysesthesias or weakness should be evaluated thoroughly. Due to impaired sensation, SCI patients may have atypical presentations of common disorders. Rotator cuff tendonitis, rotator cuff tears, subacromial bursitis, cervical radiculopathy, carpal tunnel syndrome, lateral epicondylitis, medial epicondylitis, and myofascial pain are potential pathologic entities. Less common causes of upper extremity discomfort include syringomyelia, heterotopic ossification, angina, aortic dissection and Pancoast tumors.

When prescribing a treatment plan, however, a few special issues must be addressed. The shoulder of an SCI individual is synonymous with the hip of an able-bodied person. Therefore, shoulder pain in the SCI population may have significant functional consequences. Transfers that could previously be performed independently may now require the assistance of a caregiver. If absolute or relative rest is required, a patient who was previously using a manual wheelchair may be temporarily required to use a power wheelchair. Modalities, such as ice, hot packs and ultrasound, must be prescribed with caution due to impaired sensation.

Neuropathic Pain

Neuropathic pain may be of central or peripheral origin. Patients will complain of a burning, shooting or lancing pain. The discomfort may involve the abdomen, rectum or lower extremities. It may be exacerbated by other noxious stimuli, including urinary tract infections, renal stones, HO, etc. Neuropathic pain is more common with incomplete lesions.

Neuropathic pain requires a complete assessment. Structural anatomical pathology that may be contributing to the discomfort should be identified and, if possible, treated (i.e., syrinx formation, nephrolithiasis, etc.). Although neuropathic pain is not usually responsive to acetaminophen or nonsteroidal anti-inflammatory drugs, a short trial of these medications is not unreasonable. Although frequently prescribed for neuropathic pain, tricyclic antidepressants (TCA), such as amitriptyline, imipramine and nortriptyline, should be used with caution in patients with SCI (Table 1). Tricyclic antidepressants have dose-dependent, anticholinergic side effects that may cause urinary retention, dry mouth, blurred vision, and orthostatic hypotension. In individuals with baseline orthostatic hypotension and urinary retention, these side effects may be significant. Before instituting therapy with a TCA, an EKG to exclude conduction defects should be complet-

Table 1
Medications to Treat Neuropathic Pain

Medication	Brand Name	Starting Dose	Maximum Dose	Precautions
amitriptyline	Elavil	10-25 mg qhs	150 mg qhs	anticholinergic
nortriptyline	Pamelor	10-25 mg qhs	150 mg qhs	anticholinergic
imipramine	Tofranil	10-25 mg qhs	150 mg qhs	less anticholinergic
carbamazepine	Tegretol	200 mg bid	400 mg qid	agranulocytosis, thrombocytopenia, sedation, dizziness; monitor drug levels
gabapentin	Neurontin	100 mg tid	600 mg qid	sedation, ataxia, diplopia; renal dose adjustments

ed. Anti-seizure medications, such as carbamazepine (Tegretol) and gabapentin (Neurontin), can be considered to palliate neuropathic pain in individuals with SCI.

Syringomyelia

Post-traumatic syringomyelia is a complication of SCI that may result in functional loss. This phenomenon affects approximately 5 percent of those with SCI. The incidence of syrinx may be slightly higher with tetraplegia vs. paraplegia. Syringomyelia may be recognized in acute or chronic phases of SCI. Many patients with syringomyelia, however, do not have any clinically recognizable signs or symptoms.

The pathogenesis of post-traumatic syringomyelia is not entirely understood. Cavitation of the spinal cord usually occurs at the level of the initial injury. Cavity formation may be secondary to liquefaction of the spinal cord or from the central hematoma present at the initial injury. Adhesions from arachnoiditis may exacerbate the cavity formation. The lesion usually progresses in a cephalad direction. As the lesion progresses and compromises more nerve fibers, symptoms may become more apparent. Rarely, a syrinx may extend from the cervical spinal cord into the brain stem.

Potential symptoms include increased pain and spasticity. Dysautonomic features may also be identified, such as new onset orthostatic hypotension or frank autonomic dysreflexia. In addition, some patients will experience progressive weakness, dysesthesias and hyperhidrosis. Trigeminal nerve deficit and Horner's syndrome may present if the syrinx extends into the upper cervical segments. If the lesion involves the brain stem, manifestations include hiccups, nystagmus, recurrent laryngeal nerve palsy, or death. All syringomyelia-related symptoms may be exacerbated by coughing, sneezing or body movement.

A post-traumatic syrinx is best visualized with gadolinium enhanced magnetic resonance imaging study. Radiological findings include decreased signal intensity on T1 weighted images and enhancement of the cyst. Other radiological findings include arachnoiditis, adhesions and gliosis.

Treatment of asymptomatic syrinx consists of regular surveillance of the neurological level and serial MRI studies. Surgical intervention with percutaneous drainage of the cavity or shunting of the CSF into the subarachnoid space or peritoneum may be warranted in progressive symptomatic cases. Surgical interventions may be of limited success as loculated cysts can be difficult to effectively drain and shunts may become blocked or infected. Either of these two scenarios may lead to a recurrence of syrinx formation.

Abdominal Processes

Evaluation of acute abdominal pathology in SCI patients with potentially impaired sensation can be very difficult. The typical clinical features of the acute abdomen, such as fever, guarding and rebound, may be absent. Pain, when present, may be atypical in quality and location.

Increased spasticity and a general feeling of unwellness may be the only manifestations of a surgical emergency. Cholecystitis, pancreatitis, appendicitis, gastric and duodenal ulcers, abdominal malignancies, and volvulus are some of the diagnostic possibilities. Urological causes must also be considered, including nephrolithiasis, epididymitis and testicular torsion. In women, gynecological pathology, such as ectopic pregnancy, ruptured ovarian cysts, or pelvic inflammatory diseases, can result in an acute abdomen.

When warranted, consultation with the appropriate surgical service should be obtained promptly. Not all surgical consultants have experience with SCI patients, and rehabilitation physicians may, on occasion, be required to advocate for necessary evaluations, investigations and treatments.

Hepatitis

Individuals with chronic SCI may be at increased risk for hepatitis B and C, if they were injured before 1992 and received blood products. Other risk factors include a history of intravenous drug use, multiple sexual partners, and HIV infection. In Asian-Americans, rates of hepatitis B are high. The virus is known to be transmitted by pregnant women to their children (i.e., vertical transmission). Hepatitis C is being increasingly detected. Transmission may be from household exposure. Screening for hepatitis B and C exposure is reasonable. Patients with hepatitis should be referred to a gastroenterologist for further evaluation and treatment.

Suggested Readings

Stiens SA, Johnson MC, Lyman PJ. Cardiac rehabilitation in patients with spinal cord injuries. In: Halar EH, editor. Physical medicine and rehabilitation clinics of North America: cardiac rehabilitation: part II; 1995: Vol. 6; 2:263-296.

Bach JR. Avoiding pulmonary morbidity and mortality for patients with paralytic or restrictive pulmonary syndromes. In: Bach JR, Haas F, editors. Physical medicine and rehabilitation Clinics of North America: pulmonary rehabilitation; 1996: Vol. 7; 2:423-443.

King TE, Newman K. The aging lung, chronic obstructive pulmonary disease, asthma, and pulmonary rehabilitation. In: Jahnigen D, Schrier R, editors. Geriatric medicine. 2nd edition. Malden, Ma: Blackwell Science; 1996, 643-672.

DeVivo MJ, Black KJ, Stover SL. Causes of death during the first 12 years after spinal cord injury. Archives of Physical Medicine and Rehabilitation 1993;74:248-54

Chapter 17

Wheelchair Mobility

Amy Bjornson, MPT, ATP

For most people with an SCI, a wheelchair is essential for independent mobility. In some cases, individuals may ambulate with an assistive device indoors (i.e., Canadian forearm crutches) and use a wheelchair for community mobility. Others may use a manual wheelchair (Figure 17.1) for short distances and a power wheelchair (Figure 17.4) for longer distances. Furthermore, some individuals may own two wheelchairs: one for athletic pursuits (i.e., sports wheelchair) and a wheelchair for daily activities. It is imperative to understand that, in many cases, individuals are not confined to, but liberated by, a wheelchair. Prior to prescribing this intervention, however, a thorough wheelchair assessment must be completed. Optimal wheelchair fitting requires the close cooperation of all members of the rehabilitation team.

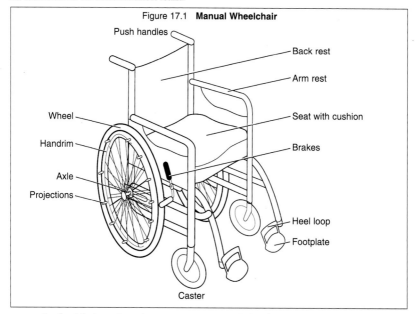

Figure 17.1 **Manual Wheelchair**

Push handles

Back rest

Arm rest

Wheel

Seat with cushion

Handrim

Brakes

Axle

Projections

Heel loop

Footplate

Caster

A wheelchair and seating system must maximize function. A properly fitted system will optimize upper extremity function and distribute seating pressure to minimize the risk of pressure ulcers. In addition, proper wheelchair fitting will minimize pelvic obliquity and concomitant scoliosis and kyphosis.

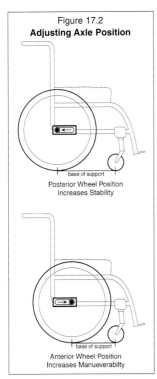

Figure 17.2
Adjusting Axle Position

base of support
Posterior Wheel Position
Increases Stability

base of support
Anterior Wheel Position
Increases Manueverabilty

Types of Wheelchairs

Wheelchairs can be self propelled (power) or propelled by the occupant (manual). Manual wheelchairs can have rigid or folding frames. Folding wheelchairs, when compared to rigid wheelchairs, are smaller, easier to transport, and less expensive. However, folding wheelchairs are heavier, less durable, and probably less energy efficient. Folding wheelchairs have more moving parts and require more frequent adjustments.

Adjusting Axle Position

By moving the wheel axle anteriorly (i.e., closer to the casters), maneuverability is increased; however, this results in decreased stability by narrowing the base of support (Figure 17.2).

Seat Height

Appropriate seat height can make transfers easier. In general, it is easiest to transfer between surfaces of similar height. Lower seat heights may allow some patients to propel their wheelchair with leg movement when the upper extremities are paralyzed. Lower seat heights will also allow for easier access under tables and desks.

Tilt and Recline

Tilt refers to movement of the seating surface relative to the floor. With tilt adjustments, however, the angle between the seat and back remain constant (i.e., no change in back angle). Increasing the "dump" is synonymous with increasing the amount of tilt. Back angle (i.e., recline) refers to the angle between the seat and back (Figure 17.3). This angle can be adjusted to accommodate patient comfort, tone, stability and function in addition to joint range of movement.

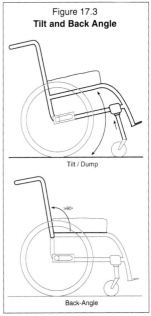

Figure 17.3
Tilt and Back Angle

Tilt / Dump

>90°

Back-Angle

Many power wheelchairs are equipped with power tilt and recline, which allow for pressure relief. Power recline is convenient for certain self-care tasks such as intermittent catheterization. Reclining, however, may result in shear forces that can contribute to pressure ulcers. Reclining can increase spasticity in some patients, as well.

Leg Rests

Adjustable leg rests are essential. Many individuals will have dependent edema that will be palliated by raising the legs. Proper lower extremity support will assist in optimal weight distribution in the buttocks and thighs. If paralyzed legs are not secured, injury may result during wheelchair mobility.

Control Mechanisms for Power Wheelchairs

Joystick: the patient uses his hand to move the joystick for wheelchair control

Head control: a specialized headrest allows the patient to drive the wheelchair

Chin control: a mini joystick, which is used to steer the wheelchair, is mounted in front of the patient's chin

Sip-and-puff: the patient pushes air through a straw, allowing for control of the wheelchair and, possibly, an environment control unit

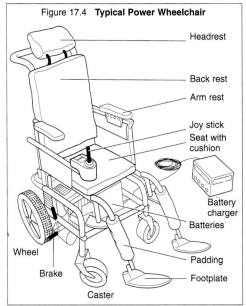

Figure 17.4 **Typical Power Wheelchair**

Headrest

Back rest

Arm rest

Joy stick

Seat with cushion

Battery charger

Batteries

Wheel

Padding

Brake

Footplate

Caster

Wheelchair Prescription Guidelines Based on Motor Level

High Tetraplegia (C2 to C4)

Power wheelchair with power tilt and/or recline
If ventilator dependent, ventilator tray
Control system depending on functional capabilities (i.e,. sip-and-puff, chin control, head control)
Excellent pressure relief seat cushion
High-back seat, headrest, trunk supports
Upper extremity support such as lap board, or arm trough

C5 Tetraplegia

Power wheelchair with power tilt and/or recline
Modified joystick or head control to operate wheelchair
Excellent pressure relief seat cushion
High-back seat, headrest, trunk supports
Upper extremity support such as lap board, or arm trough

C6 Tetraplegia

Prescribing a wheelchair for a C6 tetraplegic can be challenging. Some individuals may be able to use a manual wheelchair for all activities. Others, due to cardiovascular fitness or body weight, will require a power wheelchair for all activities. A few individuals will use a manual wheelchair for indoor short distance mobility and a power wheelchair for longer distances. With aging, pregnancy or musculoskeletal injury (e.g., rotator cuff tendonitis), a person who was initially utilizing a manual wheelchair may now require a power wheelchair.

Power Wheelchair for C6 Tetraplegia

Joystick controls
If independent in pressure relief, no need for power tilt or recline
High-back seat
Excellent pressure relief seat cushion

Manual Wheelchair for C6 Tetraplegia

Lightweight adjustable chair with solid back
Adjustable wheel position
Modified handrims (i.e., lugs or plastic coated)
Brake extensions
Excellent pressure relief cushion

C7 to T1 Tetraplegia

Lightweight manual wheelchair with solid back
Adjustable wheel position
Plastic-coated hand rims
Brake extensions
Excellent pressure relief seat cushion

T2 Paraplegia and Below

Lightweight manual wheelchair
Adjustable wheel position
Back height may be lowered due to better truncal stability
Good pressure relief seat cushion
Axle position can be placed anteriorly for improved maneuverability
Armrests may not be necessary

Seating Systems

Seating systems consist of back supports and cushions (Table 1). These systems should provide proper pressure relief, enhance truncal and pelvic stability, and provide comfort. Seating systems should be durable and should not retain perspiration or unacceptable odors.

Back supports can be made from a variety of materials. A good back support must be comfortable and should enhance truncal stability. The height of the back support is dependent on truncal stability, amount of spasticity, and level of injury.

Shower Wheelchairs

This is a special type of wheelchair that allows individuals with SCI to roll into a shower stall. It is generally used by tetraplegics. This type of chair has padded seats and allows access to the perineal areas. High tetraplegics will require a seating system with a high back, as well as tilt and/or recline capability. In addition, arm, neck and head supports may be required.

Suggested Readings

Croteau C. Wheelchair mobility. Worcester, MA: Park Press Publishing; 1998.

Fundamentals course in assistive technology. Alexandria, VA: RESNA; 1998.

Table 1 Cushion Type

CUSHION TYPE	Pressure Relief	Seating Stability	Heat Dissipation	Cleanability	Durability	Cost
Contoured foam with gel insert	GOOD	GOOD TO EXCELLENT	FAIR TO GOOD	EXCELLENT	GOOD TO EXCELLENT	HIGH
Air-filled villous	EXCELLENT	POOR TO FAIR	GOOD TO EXCELLENT	EXCELLENT	FAIR TO GOOD	HIGH
Gel-filled	GOOD	FAIR TO GOOD	EXCELLENT	EXCELLENT	FAIR	MODERATE TO HIGH
Coated contoured foam	FAIR TO GOOD	EXCELLENT	POOR TO FAIR	EXCELLENT	EXCELLENT	MODERATE TO HIGH
Foam	FAIR TO GOOD	GOOD	FAIR	POOR	FAIR TO GOOD	LOW TO MODERATE
Air-filled	FAIR	GOOD TO EXCELLENT	FAIR TO GOOD	EXCELLENT	GOOD	LOW

Reproduced with permission from Kottke FJ, Lehman JF, editors. Krusen's handbook of physical medicine and rehabilitation. 4th ed. Philadelphia: W.B. Saunders; 1990; 560.

107

Chapter 18

Environmental Modifications

Jim McCormack

Introduction

Securing an accessible apartment or house is a challenge for many persons with SCI. In some communities, the waiting period to obtain a subsidized wheelchair accessible apartment may be greater than one year. Generally, it is easier to obtain an accessible apartment if the injured person is able to pay market rent. Environmental modifications can be expensive and more difficult to perform in communities with older housing stock. If the home is rented, the cooperation of the property owner is required.

Home Modifications

Home modifications are changes to the structure of the home which allow a person with SCI to safely improve access and usability. There are a wide variety of potential home modifications and technologies available for individuals with SCI that are specific to an individual's level of injury. There are, however, some basic principles to understand. Most SCI individuals utilize a wheelchair for mobility. As a result, furniture in the home must be at an accessible height. For example, the cooking surfaces, light switches, and bed surfaces must be placed at a lower height than they are for an able-bodied person. In addition, the wheelchair must be maneuverable throughout the home, which requires wider passageways and low-resistance floors.

The nature and scope of the home modifications and technological interventions required are closely related to the level of injury. Persons with high tetraplegia, who have essentially no upper extremity function, will require the most modifications and devices. These individuals will require an environmental control system that allows for the direction of multiple daily tasks such as opening doors, turning on lights, and operating the stereo. Entrances and hallways must be wide enough to accommodate a large, power wheelchair and possibly a ventilator. Those with mid-level tetraplegia (i.e., C6) with some intact arm function may be able to perform some tasks if appropriate modifications are made. For example, modifying a standard round faucet to a lever-handled faucet may allow for more independent grooming. Individuals with lower-level tetraplegia (i.e., C8) and paraplegia will be able to manipulate objects with their hands. Consequently, fewer environmental modifications will be required.

In some cases, modifications and devices that may improve functional independence cannot be obtained due to funding limitations. Clinicians should be sensitive to budgetary issues and may assist clients in locating creative funding solutions and modification alternatives.

Home modifications of the entrance, kitchen, bathroom and bedroom are critical. They must be undertaken only after close consultation with the person with SCI, contractor, occupational therapist, physical therapist and physician. It is imperative that reputable, experienced vendors and contractors are selected.

Entrance

A proper, safe entrance is essential. It should be brightly lit so the individual can see keys and locks easily and adequately negotiate any potential irregularities in ground surface. Ideally, the entrance should be covered to offer shelter in inclement weather. If the resident utilizes a van or car, a covered garage or carport is optimal.

Outdoor Elevator

The decision to build an exterior elevator ("porch lift") instead of a ramp must be individualized. If space is limited or the height to traverse is excessive, then an elevator may be the safer choice. If a porch lift is desired, there should be an adequate landing platform (at least 30" x 40"). The control device must be at an accessible height to be usable (e.g., a joystick).

Characteristics of a Ramp

The maximum acceptable slope of a ramp is 1:12 (i.e., one foot of rise for every 12 feet of run). A less severe grade (1:20) will improve accessibility for individuals with limited endurance and upper body strength. The width of the ramp should have a minimum clearance of 36 inches. Landings at the top and bottom of the ramp should be at least 60 inches in length. If the ramp changes direction, the landing should be at least 60 square inches. If the landing is in front of a door, it should be at least 60 square inches. If a ramp has run of more than six feet, it should have handrails on both sides at a height of 32 inches from the ramp surface. It should be noted that, depending on space, these dimensions may need to be modified for private residences.

The door at the end of a ramp should be wide enough to accommodate the individual's wheelchair. An inward door swing is preferred. In addition, the resident should be able to open the door. A person with C7 tetraplegia may require door modifications (i.e., a long-lever, U-handled door), whereas an individual with C4 tetraplegia may require an electronically unlocking and mechanically opening door.

Kitchen

A well-designed kitchen will enhance the independence of a person with an SCI. Reach and maneuvering space are important. Counters and appliances should be placed to allow for the greatest degree of access throughout the kitchen. Clutter exacerbates inaccessibility and should be avoided.

One accessible work space that is at least 30 inches long for food preparation is necessary. It is important to avoid sharp projections or rough surfaces that may abrade insensate skin. Cabinets placed under the counter will be difficult to access for a person in a wheelchair. "Roll-out cabinets" and "Lazy Susan" devices will improve accessibility of stored food items.

Appliance selection should be carefully considered. The controls of ranges and cooktops should be front-mounted to prevent reaching across cooking surfaces. If there is an open area below the cooking surface, it should be well-insulated to prevent burns and electrical shock. Ovens should be self-cleaning and located next to a counter with clear floor space below it. Side-opening oven doors are desirable. Controls should be on the front of the oven. Refrigerator/freezers should be side-by-side or have at least 50 percent of the freezer space under 54 inches in height and 100 percent of the refrigerator space and the controls under 54 inches. The freezer should be self-defrosting.

Bathroom

The design of the bathroom should accommodate the individual's level of independence. The design should facilitate wheelchair maneuverability, personal grooming, and safe transfers. There should be clear approaches, properly placed grab bars, and non-slip surfaces.

The following should be considered when designing an accessible bathroom:

- To facilitate safe wheelchair-to-commode transfers, the distance between the wall and the center of the toilet seat should be 18 inches. Grab bars should be mounted on at least one side of the toilet. The toilet seat should be between 15 and 16 inches in height. Persons with some ability to stand may benefit from a slightly higher seat (17" to 19"). The toilet paper dispenser should be wall-mounted on the side wall and within easy reach. The dispenser should be installed at a maximum height of 26 inches.
- Sinks should allow for front approach. There should be 29 inches of clearance below the sink, and the minimum depth should be 19 inches. Faucets should be lever, push or electronically controlled.
- The bathing area will depend on the SCI individual's level of injury and functional capabilities. For a person with high tetraplegia, a roll-in shower is most appropriate. If bathing cannot be performed independently, then additional space should be allocated for an attendant. If the person has a lower cervical lesion or paraplegia, a tub bench may be obtained to facilitate safe transfers. A flexible hose and hand-held shower should be installed. To prevent burns, water temperature must be regulated (either at the water heater or with a thermostatic valve). Grab bars should be mounted along two sides.

Bedroom

A firm mattress at a height of 20 to 22 inches is appropriate. There should be three feet between the bed and wall to allow for level, safe transfers. A phone and alarm clock should be placed on a stand or table close to the bed. A roll-in closet with lowered clothing rods may be helpful. A "Closet Carousel" is a mechanical device that will bring items on the clothing rack to the front of the closet. This will increase convenience and accessibility.

Home Automation Devices

Home automation devices (HAD) refer to the wide range of generic environmental control devices that typically control one aspect of the environment. There are thousands of HAD in the marketplace that may assist a person with an SCI to be more independent. Examples include a remote control garage door opener, motion sensing outdoor floodlights, and automatic programmable thermostats. These devices are typically designed for able-bodied people who want to save time, energy or space. HAD sometimes require modifications to assist people with SCI in controlling the home and work environment. Many of these devices can be incorporated into new home and office construction. There are a few HAD, like motorized counter tops, that are designed specifically for people with disabilities.

Environmental Control Unit

An environmental control unit (ECU) is a tool for purposefully manipulating and interacting with the environment by accessing multiple electrical devices via technological adaptations. Unlike HAD, ECU are developed for and marketed specifically to individuals with disabilities. Each ECU product is designed to allow a person to control numerous aspects of his physical surroundings. Some issues related to selecting an ECU include the number of activities to be directed and cost. In addition, some users will require a portable unit that can be attached to the wheelchair. There are also ECU that are "stand-alone" systems, as well as systems that can be integrated with a home computer.

Two basic questions must be answered prior to purchasing an HAD or ECU. One, what part of the environment does the person want to direct (i.e., turning on lights, operating the telephone)? Two, how can the person operate the controller? Individuals with SCI may use a joystick, chin controls, sip-and-puff controls, or voice controls. Technology currently exists that allows a person to control most aspects of his environment with any part of the body capable of consistent movement. Even if this movement is minimal (e.g., the chin), the ECU can capitalize on this ability for optimal environmental control.

The manner of control (how a device is activated) is a critical consideration in the selection of ECU and HAD. The basic methods of control include direct wire, infrared, radio frequency and powerline. The direct wire method involves directly wiring an adapted switch or controller to the device to be controlled. Infrared control is built into many electronic appliances, such as a television remote, and requires a clear line of sight between the controller and the device being controlled. Radio frequency control offers wireless control without the line of sight requirement. Powerline control uses a combination of controllers and modules that plug into standard office or home AC outlets. On/off signals are sent from each controller to the device to be controlled via standard AC wiring. Unlike direct wire control, no additional wiring or modification is required with powerline control systems.

Home modifications and technological devices can improve the quality of life for persons with SCI. These can be expensive, however, and must be prescribed judiciously. It is also imperative that the person with SCI be involved in the selection and provision of any device or intervention.

Suggested Readings

Eberhardt KE. Home modifications for persons with spinal cord injury. OT Practice; 3(10):24-27.

Salmen, JP. The do able renewable home. Washington: American Association of Retired Persons.

Internet

Adaptive Environments
www.adaptenv.org

Chapter 19

Community Reintegration

Allan R. Meyers, PhD

The ultimate goal of the rehabilitation process is to reintegrate an individual with SCI into the community. The level of participation in family, vocational, avocational and civic activities is influenced by the severity of impairment (i.e., level of injury) and presence of secondary conditions (e.g., traumatic brain injury, pressure ulcer). In addition, the magnitude of financial resources, level of family supports, and scope of psychological adjustment are important. Educational and professional achievement prior to acquiring an SCI also influences community reintegration. Successful reintegration requires interventions on an individual and societal basis. For example, many people with SCI require home modifications to improve accessibility. As many people with SCI do not have the financial resources to pay for these renovations, society must provide the funds (i.e., government, foundations, charity). Furthermore, the community as a whole must have the political will to expend the financial resources to build and maintain architecturally accessible public spaces and transportation.

Community resources and assistance programs vary widely due to differing funding paradigms and eligibility criteria. As such, there is no one prescription or formula to achieve successful reintegration. Physicians must work closely with other professional colleagues (nurses, therapists, social workers and, on occasion, attorneys) as well as with the patient and his friends and family to obtain the appropriate services. This chapter will briefly address some of the issues related to reintegration.

Independent Living Centers

Independent living centers (ILC) are federally-supported, not-for-profit, consumer-governed organizations for persons with disabilities. ILC are funded at the federal level by the U.S. Department of Education's Rehabilitation Services Administration. Other financial support is derived from state and local governments, as well as by private foundations and individuals. By Congressional mandate, 50 percent of the boards of directors and employees of ILC must be persons with disabilities. At present, there are 491 ILC in the United States. The four core services provided by ILC are information and referral, skills training, peer counseling and advocacy. ILC are excellent resources for identifying and accessing community services. These centers should be contacted during the acute phase of SCI.

Income Support

As noted in chapter 1, many people with SCI were injured at a relatively young age. Many individuals had not completed their vocational training or education, or were at the beginning of their careers at the time of injury. These factors compound the challenges of obtaining paid employment. In addition, as stated in chapter 14, there are significant financial disincentives to remunerated employment.

It is estimated that 75 percent of persons with SCI are not employed; many receive income derived from public and/or private sources. Private income support is primarily in the form of commercial disability insurance benefits and, on occasion, pension benefits (i.e., the individual is "medically retired"). Some individuals may receive the proceeds of legal settlements in either structured settlements or trust income. Others receive Social Security Disability Insurance (SSDI) benefits or Supplemental Social Security Insurance (SSI) benefits. Typically, SSDI benefits are available to those who have contributed to the Social Security program for five of the past ten years prior to injury. People with SCI should apply for SSDI as early as feasible. The benefits are based on the amount of previous contributions and can be supplemented by other private income support programs or family earnings. However, if the recipient returns to paid employment, a part or all of the SSDI benefits may be eliminated.

In contrast, SSI disability benefits are available to all legal residents of the United States, including those who have never contributed to the Social Security program. SSI benefits are available to disabled persons with limited income and assets. Most states provide additional cash benefits to recipients of SSI disability benefits.

Medical Benefits

In the U.S., medical benefits are provided by pubic and private organizations (both for- and not-for-profit). People with SCI may secure benefits through private insurance, Medicaid and Medicare, or a combination of the three.

Private medical insurance is related to employment status, and many times the cost of premiums are subsidized by the employer. As noted, only a minority of persons with SCI are employed and, thereby, eligible for private coverage.

Medicaid is a state-administered medical insurance program that is primarily designed for the indigent. Funding is shared by state and federal governments and is based on a complex reimbursement formula. The breadth of services covered, level of financial reimbursement to providers, and financial eligibility criterion vary from state to state. Some states, such as Massachusetts, have relatively comprehensive coverage that includes durable medical equipment, consumable medical supplies, and personal assistant services. Other Medicaid programs have very limited benefits. Some states are encouraging, and in some cases requiring, beneficiaries to enroll in managed care programs.

Medicare is a federally-funded program. Beneficiaries include older adults (over age 65) and individuals with end-stage renal disease. Disabled persons who are unable to work permanently or for prolonged periods of time may also be eligible. Medicare consists of part A and part B. Part A does not require any premium payment and pays for inpatient hospital care, skilled nursing home services, hospice care, and home health services. The benefits are subject to co-insurance and deductibles. Part B covers most inpatient or outpatient clinician charges and outpatient diagnostic services. Part B requires the payment of a premium. In general, individuals who have received Social Security Disability benefits are eligible for Medicare benefits after a two-year waiting period. In the meantime, persons with SCI have to purchase relatively expensive private health insurance, secure Medicaid benefits, or forgo medical coverage. Some states pay for Part B benefits through the Medicaid program for those with minimal financial resources. In addition, some state Medicaid programs provide reimbursement for co-insurance and deductibles for the profoundly indigent.

Many managed care insurance programs limit choice in physicians, hospitals and other health-care providers to contain costs. Although enrolled providers in a managed care program may provide adequate choice and expertise for the otherwise well population, these restrictions can be problematic for persons with SCI. Persons with SCI have a unique set of medical issues that may not be adequately addressed by physicians, therapists and nurses inexperienced in SCI care. In addition, many private and public insurance carriers place strict (and sometimes unreasonable) restrictions on the provision of durable medical equipment (e.g., wheelchairs, tub benches, etc.). Obtaining coverage for consumable medical supplies, such as urinary catheters and latex gloves, may also be difficult. In general, private insurance carriers do not pay for personal assistant services.

The Veterans Administration (VA) operates a national network of hospitals and clinics that care for persons with SCI. VA services are available to all veterans who have served a minimum of 24 months on active duty and have been honorably discharged. VA benefits are also available to those individuals who suffered an SCI due to a service-related injury (e.g., a wartime gunshot wound).

Personal Assistant Services

Many persons with SCI require others to assist with basic personal care needs such as bathing, grooming, dressing and toileting, as well as light household tasks such as cooking and cleaning. In some cases, family members provide these services without remuneration. However, the provision of these services may distort and potentially strain family relationships.

Personal assistant services can be provided by paid personal care assistants (PCA). These services are essential for persons with SCI to live in the community, and can be provided by licensed or unlicensed individuals. In keeping with the independent living philosophy, PCA care must be directed by the person with SCI. Historically, the employer-employee relationship has been between the disabled person and the PCA. However, there are some regulatory burdens associated with employer status (e.g., withholding taxes, paying workers compensation insurance, etc.). As such, some states may provide alternate payment paradigms; for example, the state or a financial intermediary may become the employer of record and assume responsibility for compliance with appropriate employment statutes.

PCA services may be reimbursed by state Medicaid programs, workers compensation benefits, or proceeds from legal settlements. On occasion, disabled individuals may pay for services from their own financial resources. In addition, some persons with SCI provide non-cash benefits to PCA such as free room and board.

Public Transportation

Federal and state legislation mandates accessible public bus and rail transportation. These directives, however, have not been fully implemented, and it is still very difficult for a person with SCI to travel on local and regional transit systems.

Para-transit is an alternative form of public transportation. Typically, vans equipped with hydraulic lifts provide door-to-door transportation at a modest cost. To utilize services, an individual must provide some medical documentation to demonstrate eligibility. Some para-transit systems (but not all) may allow a PCA and small children to accompany the disabled person. Para-transit services may, on occasion, prioritize requests for transportation; for example, medical appointments may supersede recreational visits, and patrons who had scheduled trips may be "bumped" to provide transportation for other disabled persons.

Private transportation may be the best alternative. Lower-level tetraplegics and paraplegics should be able to drive an appropriately chosen and properly modified automobile. Many higher level tetraplegics may operate a specially modified van. The cost of a customized vehicle, however, may range from $35,000 to $50,000. Although private transportation can improve quality of life for a person with SCI, finding adequate funding remains a significant challenge.

Suggested Readings:

Hammond MC. Yes you can: a guide to self-care for persons with spinal cord injury. PVA 2nd edition; 1992.

Kaye HS. Disability Watch: The status of people with disabilities in the United States. Volcano, CA: Volcano Press, Inc; 1997.

Internet

American Disabled for Attendant Programs Today (ADAPT)
www.adapt.org

Social Security Admisistration
www.ssa.gov

Paralyzed Veterans of America
www.pva.org

Conclusion

In 1990, the U. S. Congress passed the Americans with Disabilities Act (ADA). The goal of this landmark legislation was to enable and encourage people with disabilities to fully participate in the community.

Coupled with the ADA, new medical advances and changing attitudes have helped individuals with SCI live more productive, more fulfilling lives. Research into a number of SCI-related areas continues to expand the knowledge base of this often profound impairment. As a result, this has helped caregivers to develop better medical treatments for SCI patients and rehabilitation professionals to assist these individuals in attaining their highest possible level of physical, cognitive and social functioning. Because individuals with SCI are living longer, the focus on rehabilitation has grown that much greater.

Treating a person with SCI is an excellent case study of the rehabilitation process. When initially admitted to the hospital, the patient passively receives the care and treatment of medical, nursing and allied health professionals. As the individual progresses and is transferred to the rehabilitation unit, the injured person is encouraged to depend on his own capabilities or to effectively direct the care provided by others. Finally, with community reintegration, the injured individual is less of a patient and more of a consumer of medical, social and community services.

This monograph has provided an overview of many of the major issues confronted by medical and rehabilitation professionals who work with SCI individuals. As stated in the introduction, many issues related to SCI have not been studied in a rigorous scientific manner. The contributors hope that this monograph will, in some small way, inspire researchers and caregivers of SCI individuals to continue expanding the scientific and sociomedical understanding of spinal cord injury.

Index

Tables

Illustrations

The Rehabilitation of People
with Traumatic Brain Injury

Buck H. Woo, PhD
Shanker Nesathurai, MD, FRCP(C)

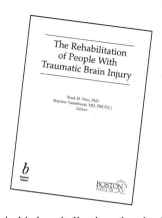

As the patient with a brain injury progresses in his hospitalization, the physiatrist is faced with coordinating the patient's rehabilitation treatment not only with acute care clinicians, but also with a variety of rehabilitation professionals. The Rehabilitation of People with Traumatic Brain Injury is a portable reference for resident physicians, therapists and other professionals interested in the treatment of patients who have sustained a traumatic brain injury. Because the nature of brain injury is a dynamic process, the monograph is organized to help conceptualize rehabilitation care along a continuum from coma to community re-entry. There are chapters on neuropharmacology, cognitive rehabilitation, behavioral management, spasticity, pediatric traumatic brain injury, and community reintegration, as well as illustrations and medication tables.

To Order: Please visit www.bumc.bu.edu/rehab
www.blacksci.co.uk/usa or contact:
Blackwell Science, Inc.
(800) 215-1000 or (781) 388-8250
Fax orders: (781) 388-8270

Other books to be published in this series include:

The Diagnosis and Management of
Bowel and Bladder Dysfunction
Essentials of Inpatient Rehabilitation
Fundamentals of Electrodiagnosis